ABC of
Multimorbidity

EDITED BY

Stewart W. Mercer

Professor of Primary Care Research
General Practice and Primary Care
Institute of Health and Wellbeing
University of Glasgow, Glasgow UK

Chris Salisbury

Professor of Primary Health Care
Centre for Academic Primary Care, NIHR School for Primary Care Research
School of Social and Community Medicine, University of Bristol, Bristol UK

Martin Fortin

Professor and Research Director
Family Medicine Department, Université de Sherbrooke
Academic Research Director, Centre de Santé et de Services Sociaux de Chicoutimi
Chicoutimi, QC, Canada

WILEY Blackwell

BMJ|Books

Library of Congress Cataloging-in-Publication Data

ABC of multimorbidity / [edited by] Stewart Mercer, Chris Salisbury, Martin Fortin.
    p.; cm.
  Includes bibliographical references and index.
  ISBN 978-1-118-38388-9 (pbk.)
  I. Mercer, Stewart, 1957- editor of compilation. II. Salisbury, Chris, editor of compilation. III. Fortin,
Martin, 1960- editor of compilation.
  [DNLM: 1. Chronic Disease. 2. Comorbidity. 3. Primary Health Care. WT 500]
  RC537
  616.85′27–dc23

                                                                                                2014003059

A catalogue record for this book is available from the British Library.

Wiley also publishes its books in a variety of electronic formats. Some content that appears in print may not be available in electronic books.

Cover image: iStockphoto.com, © 2011 Dean Mitchell
Cover design by Andy Meaden.

Set in 9.25/12 MinionPro by Laserwords Private Ltd, Chennai, India

1   2014

ABC of
Multimorbidity

ABC series

An outstanding collection of resources for everyone in primary care

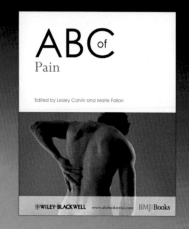
ABC of Pain
Edited by Lesley Colvin and Marie Fallon

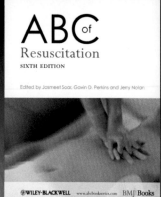
ABC of Resuscitation
SIXTH EDITION
Edited by Jasmeet Soar, Gavin D. Perkins and Jerry Nolan

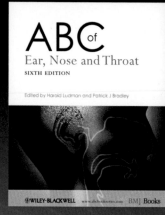
ABC of Ear, Nose and Throat
SIXTH EDITION
Edited by Harold Ludman and Patrick J Bradley

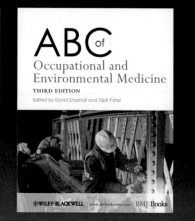
ABC of Occupational and Environmental Medicine
THIRD EDITION
Edited by David Snashall and Dipti Patel

The *ABC* series contains a wealth of indispensable resources for GPs, GP registrars, junior doctors, doctors in training and all those in primary care

▶ **Highly illustrated, informative and a practical source of knowledge**

▶ **An easy-to-use resource, covering the symptoms, investigations, treatment and management of conditions presenting in day-to-day practice and patient support**

▶ **Full colour photographs and illustrations aid diagnosis and patient understanding of a condition**

For more information on all books in the *ABC* series, including links to further information, references and links to the latest official guidelines, please visit:

www.abcbookseries.com

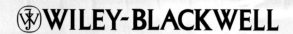

WILEY-BLACKWELL

BMJ|Books

Contents

Contributors

Marjan van den Akker
School CAPHRI, Department of Family Medicine, Institute for Education FHML, Medical Programme, Maastricht University, Maastricht, Netherlands KU Leuven, Department of General Practice, Leuven, Belgium

Elizabeth A. Bayliss
Kaiser Permanente Institute for Health Research, Department of Family Medicine, University of Colorado School of Medicine, Denver, CO, USA

Peter Bower
Centre for Primary Care, NIHR School for Primary Care Research, Manchester Academic Health Science Centre, University of Manchester, UK

Sonny Cejic
Department of Family Medicine, Schulich School of Medicine & Dentistry, The University of Western Ontario, London, ON, Canada
Byron Family Medical Centre, London, ON, Canada

Peter Coventry
NIHR CLAHRC for Greater Manchester, Manchester Academic Health Science Centre, University of Manchester, Manchester, UK

Martin Fortin
Department of Family Medicine, University of Sherbrooke, Centre for Health and Social Services Chicoutimi, Chicoutimi, QC, Canada

Katie I. Gallacher
General Practice and Primary Care, Institute of Health and Wellbeing, University of Glasgow, Glasgow, UK

Linda Gask
Centre for Primary Care, Manchester Academic Health Science Centre, University of Manchester, Manchester, UK

Jane Gunn
Department of General Practice and Primary Health Care, Academic Centre Melbourne Medical School, The University of Melbourne

Karen Kinder
Department of Health Policy and Management, Bloomberg School of Public Health, The Johns Hopkins University, Baltimore MD, USA

Frances Mair
General Practice and Primary Care, Institute of Health and Wellbeing, University of Glasgow, Glasgow, UK

Carl May
Faculty of Health Sciences, University of Southampton, Southampton, UK

Stewart W. Mercer
General Practice and Primary Care, Institute of Health and Wellbeing, University of Glasgow, Glasgow, UK

Victor M. Montori
Knowledge and Evaluation Research Unit, Department of Health Sciences Research and Medicine, Mayo Clinic, Rochester, MN, USA

Christiane Muth
Institute of General Practice, Johann Wolfgang Goethe University, Frankfurt/Main, Germany

Ignacio Ricci-Cabello
University Institute Jordi Gol Primary Care Research (IDIAP Jordi Gol), Barcelona, Spain
Autonomous University of Barcelona, Bellaterra (Cerdanyola), Spain

Martin Roland
University of Cambridge, The Primary Care Unit, Institute of Public Health, Cambridge, UK

Chris Salisbury
Centre for Academic Primary Care, NIHR School for Primary Care Research, School of Social and Community Medicine, University of Bristol, Bristol, UK

Efrat Shadmi
Faculty of Social Welfare and Health Sciences, Haifa University, Haifa, Israel

Moira Stewart
Centre for Studies in Family Medicine, Western University, Schulich School of Medicine and Dentistry, Western Centre for Public Health and Family Medicine, London, ON, Canada

Amanda L. Terry
Centre for Studies in Family Medicine, Department of Family Medicine and Department of Epidemiology & Biostatistics, Schulich School of Medicine & Dentistry, The University of Western Ontario, London, ON, Canada

Jose M. Valderas
Health Services and Policy Research Group, Department of Primary Care Health Sciences, University of Oxford, Oxford, UK
LSE Health, London School of Economics and Political Science, London, UK
University Institute Jordi Gol Primary Care Research (IDIAP Jordi Gol), Barcelona, Spain
Autonomous University of Barcelona, Bellaterra (Cerdanyola), Spain

Concepción Violán
University Institute Jordi Gol Primary Care Research (IDIAP Jordi Gol), Barcelona, Spain
Autonomous University of Barcelona, Bellaterra (Cerdanyola), Spain

Jonathan P. Weiner
Department of Health Policy and Management, Bloomberg School of Public Health, The Johns Hopkins University, Baltimore MD, USA

Preface

Clinicians and researchers from all over the world have been interested in the phenomenon of multimorbidity for more than 30 years. Interest in this topic has probably arisen because of a growing tension between two opposing developments. On the one hand, medicine is becoming ever more specialized. Attempts to improve the quality of care have led to a focus on managing care of individual long-term conditions in a very structured and standardized way. On the other hand, there is an increasing awareness that this trend may not be appropriate for people who have multimorbidity. These people are frequent users of health care, and they therefore account for a high proportion of health service contacts in both primary and secondary care. There is an increasing dissonance between the way that health services are designed and the needs of the patients that they serve.

In this book, we seek to explore some of these issues, which provide a fundamental challenge to almost every aspect of medicine from national policy about how health care should be provided to the conduct of each individual consultation between a patient and their doctor. We will discuss research on the prevalence of multimorbidity and factors associated with this. Subsequent chapters consider how multimorbidity has an impact on patients, the relationship between physical and mental health problems and how managing multiple health problems concurrently can create a heavy burden of treatment for patients. At a general practice level, we will discuss the implications of an awareness of multimorbidity for the ways in which consultations are managed, how practices are organized, the design of medical records systems and how to ensure high-quality care. At a health care system or policy level, we will provide evidence about the relationship between multimorbidity and the costs of providing care and consider the implications of multimorbidity for health policy and how health systems should be designed. Finally, we look into the future and think about how we can best improve health care in order to achieve the best possible outcomes for patients.

At the heart of this book is the authors' shared conviction that health care should be person-centred. That is, it should be designed as far as possible to understand and respond to the needs of each unique individual patient to treat people rather than diseases. This approach means that we cannot understand and manage long-term conditions in isolation. We have to understand the wider context, particularly recognizing that many patients with long-term conditions have other conditions as well and these may have important implications for management and prognosis.

Due to space limitations each chapter does not cite all references behind the chapter, but that the lead author of each chapter is happy to provide a full list of references on request.

The photographs in this book are from a public exhibition of photographs illustrating the day to day work of general practitioners in a variety of communities in Ireland. Professor Tom O'Dowd commissioned the photographer Fionn McCann to carry out the photography. We thank Trinity College Dublin for permission to use the photographs.

Stewart Mercer
Chris Salisbury
Martin Fortin

Foreword

There's nothing unusual about Albert. A patient of mine for many years, he has coronary artery disease, hypertension, hyperlipidaemia, diabetes mellitus, chronic kidney disease, osteoarthritis of the hip and – perhaps unsurprisingly – depression. His case is so typical that every General Practitioner will recognize him or have a patient with a similar selection of medical problems.

And yet whilst he is far from unusual and whilst there are more people in the UK with two or more long-term conditions than there are with one long-term condition, you would never think this was the case when you consider how so much of health care is organized.

Dealing with multimorbidity is complex, and yet most consultations, both in primary and secondary care, still have short consultations, much more appropriate for the single and straightforward. Much of the health service is organized around single conditions – look at the plethora of single-condition specialties. Look at the organization of much medical education – focused on single conditions. Look at the fragmentation of care that results. Look at the powerful impact on patients, who all too often feel as if they are treated as diseases in a person rather than a person with diseases.

Look at research, which frequently excludes patients with multiple morbidities because they make the science too complex. Look at the guidelines, which are so often focused on single conditions, mainly because they are based on the research that excluded the comorbidities. Look at the potential harms of polypharmacy. Look at the difficulty of deciding what 'good' looks like in a case like Albert's. It certainly isn't a question of treating the multiple conditions summatively – or life becomes nothing but tablets and tests.

Is it any wonder that doctors find multimorbidity complex and frequently stressful to deal with? Multimorbidity becomes a challenge for the doctor, a challenge for the patient and a challenge for the system. And in a world that talks the mantra of patient-centredness whilst frequently failing to deliver it, it becomes ever more important that we understand multimorbidity.

This book brings a wonderfully welcome, timely and important focus to this extraordinarily important topic. It may even bring a real opportunity to renew relationships between specialist and generalist doctors, who bring such different but complementary skills to our patients. Understanding multimorbidity will bring real dividends to health care. Our patients deserve nothing less.

Professor David Haslam CBE
FRCGP FRCP FFPH FAcadMed (Hon)
Chair, National Institute for Health and Care Excellence

CHAPTER 1

Introducing Multimorbidity

Martin Fortin[1], Stewart W. Mercer[2], and Chris Salisbury[3]

[1]Family Medicine Department, Université de Sherbrooke, Centre de Santé et de Services Sociaux de Chicoutimi, Canada
[2]General Practice and Primary Care, Institute of Health and Wellbeing, University of Glasgow, UK
[3]Centre for Academic Primary Care, NIHR School for Primary Care Research, School of Social and Community Medicine, University of Bristol, UK

OVERVIEW

- Multimorbidity refers to the presence of several co-occurring long-term conditions, being related or not, in a given patient
- Comorbidity refers to any additional condition that may occur during the clinical course of a patient who has an index condition that is the focus of interest
- Different terms such as frailty, disability and complexity are used by clinicians and researchers to describe conditions that are related to multimorbidity, representing different concepts
- Multimorbidity is not a medical diagnosis with well-defined criteria but represents nonetheless a major challenge for patients and clinicians, and is an emerging priority for healthcare systems.

Background

Improvements in public health and advances in the provision of health care have contributed to an increased life expectancy. People affected by medical conditions that previously led to premature death can now survive much longer. Therefore, as the population ages, an increasing number of people are now living with long-term medical conditions. Furthermore, it is now recognized that many people have *multiple* long-term conditions, a state which we refer to in this book as 'multimorbidity'.

First, we need to consider some issues of terminology and definition. The concept of multimorbidity is quite easy to understand in general terms, but quite hard to define, with many people using the same term to mean different things. Furthermore, the concept of multimorbidity is related to, but distinct from, other related terms such as comorbidity, complexity and frailty. From a medical diagnostic perspective, the terms comorbidity and multimorbidity have sometimes been used interchangeably, which is misleading. This chapter introduces the concepts of comorbidity and multimorbidity and differentiates them from other related concepts frequently used by clinicians and researchers (see Figure 1.1).

ABC of Multimorbidity, First Edition.
Edited by Stewart W. Mercer, Chris Salisbury and Martin Fortin.
© 2014 John Wiley & Sons, Ltd. Published 2014 by John Wiley & Sons, Ltd.

Box 1.1

What is the difference between multimorbidity and comorbidity?
How do the concepts of multimorbidity and frailty differ?
What are the two minimal components of a simple operational definition of multimorbidity?

Comorbidity

Feinstein, in his seminal paper published in 1970, is credited for recognizing that the therapeutic outcome of an index disease may vary depending on the type and nature of other accompanying disorders. He coined the term comorbidity: 'any distinct additional clinical entity that has existed or that may occur during the clinical course of a patient who has the index disease under study'. In the 1980s and 1990s, some authors (mostly Germans publishing articles in English) started using the word multimorbidity when referring to patients with multiple simultaneous conditions without considering any one as the index condition. The existence of other equivalent terms for multiple concurrent conditions in the medical literature (Table 1.1) has led to ambiguity and inconsistency in their use.

Multimorbidity

In 1996, van den Akker and colleagues addressed this conceptual confusion and proposed the use of two terms only: comorbidity, with the original meaning provided by Feinstein (Figure 1.1); and multimorbidity, for situations where no index condition is considered (Figures 1.1 and 1.2 represent conceptual diagrams for comorbidity and multimorbidity). Since then, many authors have adopted these terms. It should be noted that the concept of comorbidity is more relevant to specialized care within particular fields of expertise, whereas the concept of multimorbidity is more relevant to primary care and general practice settings where designating an index disease is rarely useful.

Most (but not all) authors have used the term multimorbidity to mean patients with multiple *long-term* conditions, while others (most notably Barbara Starfield) have suggested that acute conditions should not be ignored. However, restricting the definition to long-term conditions is more useful for most purposes,

Table 1.1 Terms used to designate multiple conditions.

Comorbidity
Multimorbidity
Multi-morbidity
Polymorbidity
Poly-morbidity
Polymorbidities
Polypathology
Poly-pathology
Polypathologies
Pluripathology
Multipathology
Multi-pathology
Multipathologies

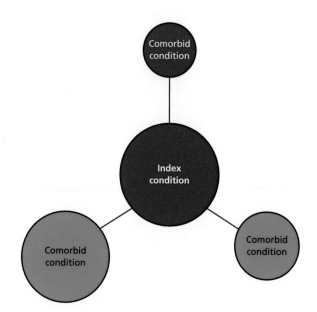

Figure 1.1 Conceptual diagram of comorbidity. Adapted from: Boyd CM and Fortin M. 2011.

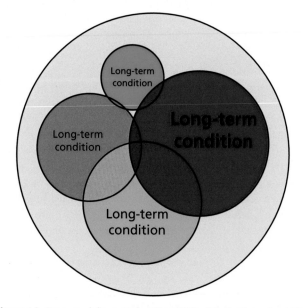

Figure 1.2 Conceptual diagram of multimorbidity. Adapted from: Boyd CM and Fortin M. 2011.

because it the fact that conditions endure over a prolonged period that leads to the accumulation of problems in one individual. In the context of multimorbidity, the definition of a long-term or chronic condition is not straightforward. Time intervals of 3, 6 and 12 months have been used to define 'long-term' conditions. The World Health Organization has defined chronic condition as a health problem that requires ongoing management over a period of years or decades. At the very least, most people probably agree that a condition that lasts more than one year and requires ongoing medical care is a long-term condition. It is convenient at this point to specify that the term health condition is usually used in this context as it is more encompassing and less restrictive than terms such as disease (generally manifested by signs and symptoms) or illness (which also refers to a person's perception of his or her health).

Other related concepts

Recognizing the presence of multimorbidity in a patient may lead to uncovering other challenging problems, not always well defined, but generally considered to be closely related to the presence of multiple diseases. These problems include concepts such as disability, frailty and patient complexity. Disability can be defined as a difficulty or dependency in carrying out activities that are essential for an independent living. Frailty represents a state of increased vulnerability to stressors that results from decreased physiologic reserves of multiple physiological systems, bearing a similarity with disability in associated outcomes. Patient complexity, although intuitively understood, is a multifaceted concept in which medical, social and behavioural factors play a role. All these concepts are more common in patients with multimorbidity and complicate the management of patients but are distinct from multimorbidity.

Other aspects related to the presence of multiple long-term conditions such as potential aetiological associations (where two conditions are caused by the same underlying factor), direct causation (where one condition causes a second condition) and correlation of associated risk factors with multimorbidity also has an impact on the management of patients.

Multimorbidity: clinical versus operational definition

Multimorbidity is not a medical diagnosis with well-defined criteria. It is rather a state by which the clinician along with the patient and/or the family faces the multiplicity of long-term conditions experienced by the patient. This represents the **clinical definition** of multimorbidity. In this respect and on clinical grounds, there is no clear number of conditions for which the patient is considered 'multimorbid'. The cut-off may vary from one patient to another or between one clinician and another depending on many factors. Other states share the same imprecision, for example being old or frail. However, for the purposes of research and reporting, we need to agree on a definition that is measurable, comparable and conceptually sound. Various definitions are used in the literature,

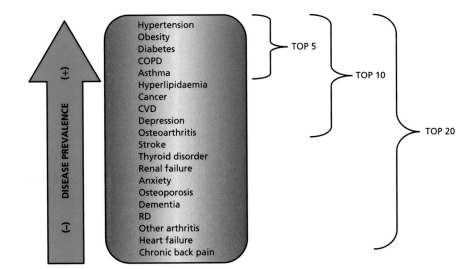

Figure 1.3 Diagram illustrating different cut-off points for the number of conditions taken into account: COPD, chronic obstructive pulmonary disease; CVD, cardiovascular disease and RD, rheumatic disease.

but many publications on multimorbidity lack clarity in the definition used.

A simple operational definition of multimorbidity includes at least two components: (1) the minimum number of conditions considered to be classified as 'multimorbidity' and (2) the conditions taken into account. In regard to the minimum number of conditions considered, the co-occurrence of two or more conditions is the **operational definition** most frequently used in the medical literature. However, cut-off counts of three, four and five long-term conditions have also been used or suggested by different authors. This distinction is important for reporting on the epidemiology of multimorbidity. But for clinical purposes, most doctors think of multimorbidity as referring to patients with multiple long-term conditions, without referring to a specific number.

The list of long-term conditions that have been taken into account in different studies on multimorbidity so far has varied greatly. Some authors have limited their investigation to a short list of conditions, ignoring all the other conditions a patient may have had. Others have included all possible long-term conditions experienced by the patient. This factor has an important impact on studies of the prevalence of multimorbidity (see Chapter 2). Not surprisingly, the longer the list of long-term conditions considered, the higher the probability of detecting the presence of multimorbidity. In reference to the type of conditions taken into account, the most prevalent chronic conditions with a high impact or burden on a given population should be included. Figure 1.3 presents a list of long-term conditions based on their frequency. From this we can imagine the impact of limiting the investigation to the top 5 or top 10 long-term conditions. For example, a patient with hypertension, renal failure, heart failure and osteoporosis would not be considered as a case of multimorbidity if we limit the investigation to the top 10! As a compromise to allow for good estimates in population prevalence studies, some authors have suggested the use of a minimal list of the 12 more frequent long-term conditions in a given context or setting. However, on clinical grounds and for a given patient, all long-term conditions should be considered.

Clinical vignettes illustrating typical cases of multimorbidity in relationship with the other overlapping concepts of complexity and comorbidity are presented in Boxes 1.2–1.4.

Box 1.2 **Multimorbidity**

Mrs. MM, 48 years old

Mrs. MM is married and a mother of three teenagers. She works as a teacher in an elementary school. She is obese and being treated for hypertension and asthma, but her main concern is related to her recurrent depression for which she has been put on anti-depressant therapy for life. She does not exercise very often as she is symptomatic of a hip bursitis that has responded neither to medication nor to physical therapy. In the last 6 months, she has been bothered by symptoms of perimenopause with frequent hot flashes. She has been offered hormone therapy but she is uncertain about accepting as her mother died from breast cancer 2 years ago.

With at least six chronic conditions requiring management, Mrs. MM's overall condition can be considered as multimorbidity.

Box 1.3 **Multimorbidity and complexity**

Mr. MC, 60 years old

Mr. MC, a man living in poverty, has been suffering from chronic obstructive pulmonary disease since 10 years. He has just been discharged from the hospital following a complicated pneumonia that required 3 days of respiratory support in the intensive care unit. He is now back home in his small flat in a disadvantaged neighbourhood downtown. Living alone with no family visiting, he receives support from community health services. He is a heavy drinker and does not cooperate well with caregivers. Living on welfare assistance, most of his money is spent on cigarettes and alcohol. He has had two previous surgeries for peripheral arterial insufficiency. His chronic kidney failure is worsening over time. With two episodes of gastritis accompanied by haemorrhaging in the past year, he has been prescribed proton pump inhibitors on a regular basis. He rarely shows up for his medical appointments with either his medical doctor or specialists. He is back in the hospital when things go wrong. He has been hospitalized four times a year over the past 3 years including two stays in a psychiatric ward for mental confusion and bizarre behaviour.

With at least five long-term conditions and the associated social and behavioural factors, Mr. MC's condition can be classified as complexity or complex multimorbidity.

Box 1.4 **Multimorbidity and comorbidity**

Mr. CO, 57 years old

Mr. CO, 57 years old, was diagnosed with type-2 diabetes at the age of 42. Recurrent leg ulcers and vascular insufficiency have led to an amputation of his left leg below the knee following several unsuccessful surgeries. He has had a first myocardial infarction at the age of 50 and is still inconvenienced by recurring symptoms of angina requiring nitroglycerine. Treated for hyperlipidaemia and hypertension, Mr. CO is compliant with the medication he was prescribed to take daily. Last year, Mr. CO suffered from a zoster on the upper part of the abdomen that left him with chronic pain requiring medication on a regular basis. Mr. CO is also concerned with the recent onset of erectile dysfunction. Mr. CO is under the care of a family doctor and several specialists. He is well supported by an understanding wife. He is the owner of a small business for which he is still doing administrative work.

Mr. CO can be classified as a case of diabetes with comorbidity. His diabetes is considered as the index disease. However, from a generalist perspective, Mr. CO is also a case of multimorbidity.

Severity

This chapter would not be complete without saying a word about severity. Not all conditions have the same severity. Some long-term conditions are relatively mild compared to other conditions in terms of their impact on the patient. For example, treated hypothyroidism could be considered less severe than diabetes but both could be considered as long-term chronic conditions. Some conditions (such as hypertension) may not cause any symptoms for the patient but still have potentially severe consequences. In addition, for any given condition, level of severity may vary from one patient to another. For example, psoriasis can be a minor and occasional nuisance for some patients but have a life-changing impact on others. These variations in severity between conditions and between individuals are rarely taken into account in reporting on multimorbidity. These factors are however important for clinicians as they may guide the decision-making process with a particular patient.

Measures

Various measures of comorbidity or multimorbidity have been used in the literature, but so far no consensus exists on which ones could or should be used in the clinical context. Their use is mainly limited to research. Some are more relevant to the primary care context as they relate well with issues of interest such as quality of life and psychological distress. Universal use of the electronic medical record, however, may bring some opportunity to develop and use such an index for clinical purposes.

Multimorbidity as an emerging priority

This discussion about the definition of multimorbidity may appear a little academic but some points are clear. Multimorbidity is widespread and increasingly common as the population gets older. Multimorbidity has many and various impacts on patients and can make their life very complicated. Multimorbidity often results in chaotic care trajectories and contributes to an increase in utilization of healthcare resources.

Multimorbidity calls for a special attention from care providers. It is very important to consider the implications of multimorbidity in how health care is planned and provided. This book will discuss these issues in more detail.

Further reading

Boyd, C. & Fortin, M. (2011) Future of multimorbidity research: how should understanding of multimorbidity should inform health system design. *Public Health Reviews*, **32–32**, 451–474.

Fortin, M., Stewart, M., Poitras, M.-E., Almirall, J. & Maddocks, H. (2012) A systematic review of prevalence studies on multimorbidity: toward a more uniform methodology. *Annals of Family Medicine*, **10**, 142–151.

Fried, L.P., Ferrucci, L., Darer, J., Williamson, J.D. & Anderson, G. (2004) Untangling the concepts of disability, frailty, and comorbidity: implications for improved targeting and care. *Journals of Gerontology. Series A, Biological Sciences and Medical Sciences*, **59**, 255–263.

Grant, R.W., Ashburner, J.M., Hong, C.C., Chang, Y., Barry, M.J. & Atlas, S.J. (2011) Defining patient complexity from the primary care physician's perspective: a cohort study. *Annals of Internal Medicine*, **155**, 797–804.

Valderas, J.M., Starfield, B., Sibbald, B., Salisbury, C. & Roland, M. (2009) Defining comorbidity: implications for understanding health and health services. *Annals of Family Medicine*, **7**, 357–363.

van den Akker, M., Buntinx, F. & Knottnerus, J.A. (1996) Comorbidity or multimorbidity: what's in a name? A review of literature. *The European Journal of General Practice*, **2**, 65–70.

CHAPTER 2

How Common Is Multimorbidity?

Marjan van den Akker[1,2] *and Christiane Muth*[3]

[1]School CAPHRI, Department of Family Medicine, Institute for Education FHML, Medical Programme, Maastricht University, Netherlands
[2]Department of General Practice, KU Leuven, Belgium
[3]Institute of General Practice, Johann Wolfgang Goethe University, Germany

---

OVERVIEW

- The absolute number of patients suffering from multimorbidity – however, wherever and whenever measured – is large and increasing
- The absolute number of people with multimorbidity is higher among young and middle-aged people (<65 years) than among older people (≥ 65 years)
- Multimorbidity is more frequent among older patients and patients with lower socio-economic status
- Patients suffering from multimorbidity are at risk of fragmented care and polypharmacy
- Further characterization of patients with multimorbidity in terms of both disease profiles and psychosocial profiles is warranted, in order to develop better patient-oriented care programmes and clinical decision support.

Box 2.1

Are there big differences between the prevalence of multimorbidity in non-western countries as compared to developed countries?
What are the two factors that have the strongest association with the prevalence of multimorbidity?
What is a possible explanation for the plateau that is observed at an advanced age in prevalence studies?
How is polypharmacy defined?

Introduction

In Chapter 1, the multiplicity and complexity of the concept of multimorbidity was introduced. Differing concepts and definitions of multimorbidity have led to a variety of ways of measuring multimorbidity. Applying these in different settings and populations and making use of different data sources mean that prevalence estimates vary widely and are not easy to compare and interpret. In this chapter, we will present estimates of prevalence rates of multimorbidity in different settings and using different definitions. In 'Prevalence estimates' section, we will discuss socio-economic influences as well as biopsychosocial parameters, which are known to be associated with an increased prevalence of multimorbidity, for example the influence of social class or social network and cross-country differences. In 'Factors associated with the prevalence of multimorbidity' section, some insight is provided into the problem of polypharmacy – one of the most prominent consequences of multimorbidity (Box 2.1).

Prevalence estimates

The setting of studies assessing the prevalence of multimorbidity influences the findings. As can be expected, there are large differences in the prevalence of multimorbidity between older patients in hospital and those consulting in primary care and community-dwelling older people. Looking at hospitalized patients, they often suffer from multiple chronic diseases. Studies from different Western countries report prevalence rates of 22–65% multimorbidity for all inpatients, and even up to 96% in patients admitted from an emergency unit to the medical wards.

The prevalence of multimorbidity in primary care and general populations also varies widely across studies in Western countries. In some countries those populations are very similar, whereas in other countries not all inhabitants are enrolled in primary care. An average prevalence of multimorbidity of 20–30% has been reported when considering the whole population, and 55–98% when only older people are included in the analyses. Looking at different (cross-sectional) studies, both higher prevalence and lower prevalence are reported in the literature. As pointed out in Chapter 1, the methodology used has a strong influence on the prevalence of multimorbidity found. However, the proportions are reasonably comparable if only studies are included that measure multimorbidity in a set of 12 or more diseases (Figure 2.1).

Several studies have indicated an increase in multimorbidity prevalence during the first decade of this century, suggesting a likely further rise of multimorbidity prevalence in the coming years.

Also in non-Western countries such as India, Bangladesh and Brazil, high prevalence of multimorbidity, similar to those in developed countries, is found. For people aged 60 and older in

ABC of Multimorbidity, First Edition.
Edited by Stewart W. Mercer, Chris Salisbury and Martin Fortin.
© 2014 John Wiley & Sons, Ltd. Published 2014 by John Wiley & Sons, Ltd.

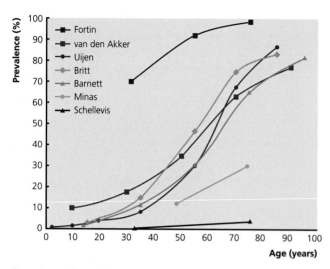

Figure 2.1 Multimorbidity reported in primary care settings.

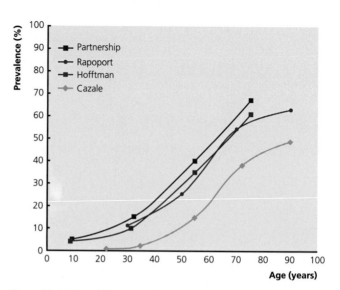

Figure 2.2 Multimorbidity reported in the general population.

the northern India, a prevalence of 83% was reported, whereas the prevalence reported in Bangladesh in the same age group was 54%. In a Brazilian population, somatic and mental disorders were found to co-occur frequently, suggesting that substantial proportions of all morbidities in the community are not attributable to disorder-specific risks but rather to a few generic liability factors applicable to many disorders, including both chronic medical and psychiatric disorders. For developing countries, the prevalence of multimorbidity may also be expected to rise further, as the life expectancy continues to increase chronic diseases become more frequent.

Multimorbidity has many consequences and it is related to greater use of healthcare services. The high prevalence of multimorbidity thus results in more frequent consultations; in general practice, most consultations – up to as much as 80% – concern patients with multimorbidity. To inform clinicians, researchers and policy makers, knowledge about frequent combinations of diseases – the so-called clusters or patterns of multimorbidity – is essential, given that there are about 10 000 recognized single diseases and the resulting quantity of potential combinations. Therefore, attention on clusters of co-occurring diseases is increasing. Clusters reported in different populations are cardiovascular/metabolic; anxiety/depression/psychological diseases; and neuropsychiatric or psychogeriatric clustering. Several other patterns have been observed in single studies, but have not yet been confirmed by others.

Factors associated with the prevalence of multimorbidity

In spite of the variability, all studies agree that the prevalence of multimorbidity in older populations is much higher than the prevalence of even the most common single diseases among older patients, such as heart failure and arthritis. Furthermore, in all studies, age is reported to be one of the major risk factors for multimorbidity, which is often positioned as a condition of older patients. However, it is increasingly recognized that the absolute number of patients suffering from multimorbidity is highest among those aged less than 65: of all people with multimorbidity, up to

70% people have been reported to be below 65 years. One should keep in mind, though, that on average multimorbidity may be more complex in older patients than in younger patients because of a higher number of co-occurring diseases. For example, in a nursing home sample, a mean of 17 chronic diseases per patient has been reported. One can see an S-shape curve with a serious rise of the prevalence of multimorbidity starting around the age of 40 and a plateau around the age of 70, both in a primary care population and in the general population (Figure 2.2).

This observed phenomenon could have different meanings, as the data from cross-sectional studies do not allow a longitudinal interpretation. The most likely interpretation is that the plateau effect is due to the increased mortality among people with multimorbidity in comparison to people without multimorbidity, so that the relative rate of multimorbidity tends to decrease. If so, this is a call for an early identification of multimorbidity in order to try to limit further worsening of the patients' conditions, but more longitudinal studies are needed.

Consistently, across studies, older patients and people from lower social classes are more likely to be affected by multimorbidity. This has been shown whether lower socio-economic status has been measured as financial hardships during childhood, low income during adulthood, a lower educational level or a lower level of health literacy. Also a higher level of deprivation in the area where people live has been shown to be associated with a higher prevalence. Not only people with lower socio-economic status are found to have an increased risk of multimorbidity, they also develop it much earlier in life – up to 15 years – as compared to that of their affluent counterparts (Figure 2.3).

This social gradient was also found to be associated with the presence of mental health disorders, particularly depression (Figure 2.4).

Less consistently, women have been reported to have a higher prevalence of multimorbidity compared with that of men. Other risk factors – although studied scarcely – include mental health problems and a high external health locus of control. Some studies suggest that a high internal health locus of control and factors such

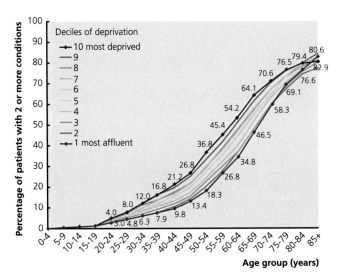

Figure 2.3 Prevalence of multimorbidity by age and socioeconomic status. On socioeconomic status scale, 1 = most affluent and 10 = most deprived. Source: Barnett *et al.* 2012. Reproduced with permission of Elsevier.

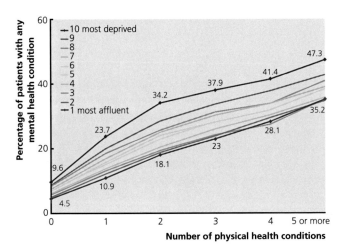

Figure 2.4 Physical and mental health comorbidity and the association with socioeconomic status. On socioeconomic status scale, 1 = most affluent and 10 = most deprived. Source: Barnett *et al.* 2012. Reproduced with permission of Elsevier.

as a larger social network and living with a family might be seen as protective factors. Other psychosocial factors that are related to serious outcomes (e.g. increased mortality), such as loneliness and cognitive status, have not as yet been found to be related to an increased risk for multimorbidity.

From multimorbidity to polypharmacy

Dealing with patients with multimorbidity frequently results in the prescription of multiple medications - also known as polypharmacy. Polypharmacy, often defined as the simultaneous use of five or more chronic medications, affects almost two-thirds of the people at the age of 70 or older - about one-third of this age group takes nine or more drugs each day. The prevalence and

predictors of polypharmacy have been analyzed in many studies. Multimorbidity is one of the strongest predictors of polypharmacy, and also specific chronic diseases such as hypertension, coronary heart disease, heart failure, Chronic obstructive pulmonary disease (COPD), chronic renal failure and diabetes mellitus are predictors of polypharmacy. Multiple drugs are prescribed for the treatment of each of these individual diseases. Moreover, the vast majority of patients with conditions such as chronic heart failure suffer from multimorbidity.

Polypharmacy brings additional risks to patients with multimorbidity: a higher chance of adverse drug reactions (ADRs) and related events – especially in older patients and those with a larger number of prescriptions – and also the risk of under treatment. An estimated rate of about 6.5% of all hospitalizations – about half of them preventable – is caused by ADRs, of which more than one-third are considered to be serious, about 2% of them are even deadly and all are costly. Preventable cases are often associated with inappropriate prescriptions, but also a lack of patient adherence causes about one-fifth. It has clearly been shown that a higher number of medications or a more complex medication regimen have a negative influence on patients' adherence in general – both on taking medications and on adherence with medical appointments.

Vertically organized care chains that are in accordance with disease-oriented guidelines and disease-specific care management programmes may exaggerate these problems and may hamper good quality of care (see also Chapters 5 and 6). Driving factors in polypharmacy include an uncritical use of multiple guidelines in patients with multimorbidity; fragmentation of care, such as care by different specialists; and hospital systems that are not integrated with primary care. Also, patients with multimorbidity often feel overwhelmed as they have to manage their burden of both their diseases and treatments. There has been a call to specifically pay attention to these patients' treatment burden using a so-called minimally disruptive medicine approach, where treatment regimens should be adapted to patients' daily lives (see Chapter 8). The high prevalence and impact of multimorbidity is clear, but much less is known about the factors related to the occurrence of multimorbidity. Given the large societal impact of multimorbidity, further profiling and monitoring of patients at risk is needed.

Further reading

Agborsangaya, C.B., Lau, D., Lahtinen, M. *et al.* (2012) Multimorbidity prevalence and patterns across socioeconomic determinants: a cross-sectional survey. *BMC Public Health*, **12**, 201.

Barnett, K., Mercer, S., M, N. *et al.* (2012) Epidemiology of multimorbidity and implications for health care, research, and medical edication: a cross-sectional study. *Lancet*, **379, 380** (9836), 37–43.

Fortin, M., Stewart, M., Poitras, M.E. *et al.* (2012) A systematic review of prevalence studies on multimorbidity: toward a more uniform methodology. *Annals of Family Medicine*, **10** (2), 142–151.

France, E.F., Wyke, S., Gunn, J.M. *et al.* (2012) Multimorbidity in primary care: a systematic review of prospective cohort studies. *British Journal of General Practice*, **62** (597), e297–307.

Tucker-Seeley, R., Li, Y. *et al.* (2011) Lifecourse socioeconomic circumstances and multimorbidity among older adults. *BMC Public Health*, **11**, 313.

A complete overview of references used is available from the authors.

CHAPTER 3

How Does Multimorbidity Affect Patients?

Elizabeth A. Bayliss

Kaiser Permanente Institute for Health Research, Department of Family Medicine, University of Colorado School of Medicine, USA

OVERVIEW

- Greater morbidity burden can be associated with lower quality of life, lower physical function and poor emotional well-being
- Highly symptomatic conditions that affect quality of life for patients are highly prevalent; however, clinical care and biomedical research tend to prioritize treatment of conditions that increase mortality and resource use
- Assessing and understanding patient's perceptions and priorities are important for planning care for populations and for individuals
- Multimorbidity management should focus on maximizing self-care potential, supporting patients (and their caregivers) and insuring good care coordination and continuity of care.

Box 3.1

What are the main patient-perceived outcomes associated with greater morbidity burden?
What kind of multimorbidity measures are more appropriate to accurately assess symptom burden?
What kind of multimorbidity measures are more appropriate to accurately predict mortality, cost or care and hospitalization?

Background

Multimorbidity affects all aspects of patients' lives. People with multimorbidity have more requirements for health care – including visits to health professionals, hospitalizations and use of emergency services. Having multiple conditions increases patients' risk of disability, causes more physical limitations and affects individuals' ability to care for themselves. Quality of life (QOL), emotional well-being and social interactions may also be affected. People with multimorbidity are less likely to be employed to contribute economically on a personal level and on a societal level. However, not all persons with multimorbidity experience adverse effects: certain combinations of conditions have greater effects than others; and patients have a range of personal, social and societal resources to draw upon for self-care.

Perceptions of multimorbidity

Morbidity burden is in the eye of the beholder. While patients are likely to define multimorbidity in terms of conditions and symptoms that affect function, clinicians are likely to refer to coexisting

diseases. Patients may describe functional limitations such as back pain plus shortness of breath, while clinicians may be concerned about the long-term effects of hypertension and hyperlipidaemia on renal function. Making care decisions requires understanding and incorporating varying perspectives.

On a population level, specific measures of morbidity establish associations between morbidity burden and patient outcomes. It is necessary to use appropriate measures to accurately assess the effects of morbidity burden on patients. Measures that incorporate patient input are more likely to give an accurate assessment of symptom burden; while measures that are based on diagnosis codes and other objective data are more likely to give an accurate assessment of mortality risk, cost of care, risk of hospitalization and other more objective outcomes (Figure 3.1). It is clear that multimorbidity, in general, is associated with increased mortality, higher rates of hospitalization, decrease in functional status, increased financial burdens of medical care and lower quality of life (Box 3.1).

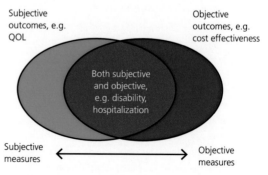

Figure 3.1 Different measures are associated with different outcomes.

ABC of Multimorbidity, First Edition.
Edited by Stewart W. Mercer, Chris Salisbury and Martin Fortin.
© 2014 John Wiley & Sons, Ltd. Published 2014 by John Wiley & Sons, Ltd.

Mortality and hospitalization

Although the simplest proxy for degree of morbidity is age (with older age associated with more multimorbidity), having more coexisting chronic conditions is associated with higher rates of mortality that is independent of age. Within populations of people with multimorbidity, mortality is higher among subgroups characterized by certain chronic conditions such as congestive heart failure, cancer, chronic lung disease, and advanced hepatic and renal diseases. Although more multimorbidity is clearly associated with lower socio-economic status that is associated with mortality, it is unclear whether the association between morbidity and mortality is greater in groups characterized by low socio-economic status.

Risk of hospitalization follows similar patterns. People with multimorbidity are more likely to be hospitalized for a range of conditions than those with no chronic conditions – independent of age group and in populations of all ages. Mental as well as physical comorbidities affect hospitalization, although diseases of circulatory, respiratory and metabolic systems and oncology are particularly influential. Hospitalizations can also result from complications of treating multiple conditions such as adverse drug reactions and medical errors.

Functional status and quality of life

Overall, greater multimorbidity is associated with lower reported physical well-being and lower functional status. In contrast to multimorbidity associated with mortality and hospitalization, coexisting conditions that limit physical functioning tend to be those that are highly prevalent and most symptomatic to patients, such as back pain, obesity, arthritis, visual impairments and chronic cardiopulmonary disease. Mental illness as a comorbidity also has a consistently negative effect and likely interacts with other conditions to affect functional status. A subset of symptomatic conditions (musculoskeletal, hearing, vision, diabetes or depression) are specifically associated with work limitations – which may affect patients' economic well-being as well as their physical quality of life. Low functional status because of multimorbidity may also affect friends and family members who act as either formal or informal caregivers for patients. Care for individuals with functional limitations is usually uncompensated and are difficult to quantify, but is of a far greater magnitude on a population level than formal caregiving (Figure 3.2).

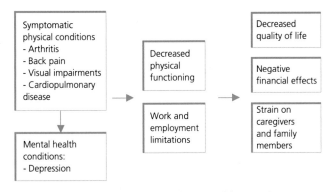

Figure 3.2 Example causes and effects of decreased functional status because of multimorbidity.

As chronic conditions increase in severity and number, they have a greater effect on QOL in general. In addition to physical functioning, QOL is also a function of age, emotional well-being, population and cultural norms, and social support, among other factors. Greater multimorbidity of physical conditions is associated with a lower emotional well-being and a greater risk of depression, and this is especially true for populations with painful physical symptoms. And in populations with multiple chronic medical conditions, depression contributes to mental functioning, disability and quality of life.

The effect of multimorbidity on various domains of QOL is nonlinear and age dependent: an initial condition may have a substantial effect on self-rated health in some age groups; and in all age groups having approximately four or more conditions appears to particularly affect physical functioning and emotional well-being. The effect of multimorbidity on QOL is further moderated by variable adaptation to the effects of total disease burden. Individuals with low self-efficacy, poor problem-solving skills and less social support and with higher degrees of helplessness appear to experience more negative effects of multimorbidity on QOL.

Thus, supporting patient characteristics that improve self-care and physical and emotional functioning may improve QOL for individuals with multimorbidity. Interventions to promote self-efficacy, improve problem-solving approaches to illness, treat depressive disorders, provide adequate pain management for musculoskeletal conditions and maximize social support should be explored for all eligible patients.

Patient experiences

Townsend et al. (2003) found that patients' ' ... experience of multiple morbidity [is] characterized by fluctuating symptoms, fear, uncertainty and lack of control'. They report barriers to the care process that reflect the magnitude of their disease burden – and perceived barriers increase with the level of morbidity.

Patient-reported barriers to self-management include financial constraints, having symptoms and treatments that interfere with each other, physical limitations, 'hassles' with interacting with the healthcare system, decreased medication adherence and a need to prioritize care (Box 3.2).

Multimorbidity requires attention to the collaborative care needs of patients and clinicians. Interactions with the healthcare system are particularly problematic. People with multimorbidity may see numerous different doctors and nurses over the course of a year, and doctors treating multimorbid populations may address several different problems at each visit. This may result in miscommunications and conflicting messages to patients. Patients may also receive conflicting information from different healthcare providers and experience unnecessary or duplicative tests. Unsurprisingly, this can result in lower patient-reported ratings of communication – even for concordant conditions with similar management strategies. One result of miscommunication is that patients with greater multimorbidity may feel that they are obtaining lower quality care (Shadmi et al., 2006).

This frustration is mirrored by clinicians, who struggle with prioritizing the healthcare demands of patients with multimorbidity

Box 3.2 **Patient vignette**

I take quite a few pills, quite a bit of medication, but I have that all laid out at home. I put a week's supply out once a week so I know when to take my pills. Some of them I take in the morning, some of them in the afternoon or early afternoon and then a few at night when I am ready to go to bed … my basic problems are diabetes and heart … and high blood pressure of course. What else? Arthritis. I elevate my legs to take care of the arthritis in the knees because they tell me that it is the changing weather … I try to watch my diet … the single thing that bothers me the most is my diminished capacity to do things that I particularly enjoy doing – a lot now depends on my wife … I think the primary concern I have got is weight management. I managed to lose over 30 pounds after my heart surgery … and I have gained it all back … that was before I started on insulin … I used to bike around the neighbourhood, but one of the things that I have lost is balance … and I could not do much in the way of walking, because of the sciatica … and I have had a little bit of diabetes haemorrhaging in my left eye which bothers me … so arthritis in my knees and ankles and back is the most troublesome … and I am not tolerant of the opiate family of drugs at all – I itch like crazy – so acetaminophen is my primary pain medication … It actually has no impact on my work since I am punching my keyboard and talking on the phone … and as long as I can be productive I want to work.

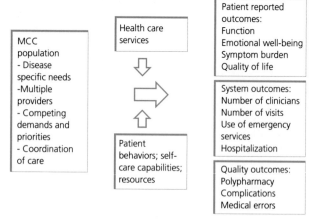

Figure 3.3 Example outcomes relevant to persons with multimorbidity.

and acknowledge the inconveniences of approaching individual chronic conditions in sequence (Bower *et al.*, 2011). Using technology to improve informational continuity between providers has the potential to alleviate conflicting messages and avoid duplicating tests, and maximizing interpersonal continuity can facilitate goal setting and communication.

Patients with multimorbidity report competing demands between care requirements for different chronic conditions, and between social and personal demands and chronic disease management. However, perceptions of disease importance and competing demands vary by demographic group and cultural background. One group with diabetes and comorbid conditions may be more likely to place a lower priority on their diabetes and have worse diabetes self-management abilities; while another group may report diabetes and arthritis as primary sources of concern. Polypharmacy creates an additional set of competing demands with varying dosing schedules, side effects and financial burden.

To improve care for the multimorbid population, it is important that investigations and interventions address multimorbidity, specifically the study outcomes that are important to patients. Outcomes have already been developed that assess quality of life, functional status, symptom burden and emotional well-being. Additional system-level outcomes address healthcare burden, polypharmacy, and use of healthcare services such as hospitalization or office visits. However, there is much room for improvement in developing other outcomes that will inform better care for this population. These might include outcomes that reflect quality of care such as complication rates, overuse of procedures and successful care coordination, among others. Figure 3.3 illustrates examples of outcomes that may contribute to patient-centred guidelines for multimorbidity care.

Adaptive strategies

Well-established self-care behaviours for 'routine' chronic conditions may provide some relief for patients in the face of significant competing demands. Persons with high levels of medication adherence or good chronic disease control (for diabetes, hypertension and hyperlipidaemia) are likely to maintain these patterns even when faced with a new chronic disease diagnoses. This suggests that (a) competing demands may reflect unclear prioritization; and (b) well-established routines along with sufficient knowledge about self-care may decrease the burden of self-care for persons with multiple chronic conditions. Patients have emphasized the need for care processes that are patient-centred, individualized and flexible enough to meet the care demands of juggling multiple conditions. They would like clinicians to appreciate that each person has unique needs, and that these needs are likely to fluctuate. Patients, clinicians and healthcare systems agree that support from a single coordinator of care may help patients prioritize their competing demands (Box 3.3).

Box 3.3 **Principles of multimorbidity management:**

Maximize self-care potential

– Knowledge and skills
– Self-efficacy
– Social support
– Address limiting symptoms (pain and mood)
– Simplify polypharmacy
– Evaluate financial barriers to care

Coordinate care

– Jointly prioritize care processes and goals (shared decision-making)
– Informational continuity (provider–provider)
– Single contact point for patients and interpersonal continuity (patient–provider)

Further reading

Bayliss, E.A., Edwards, A.E., Steiner, J.F. & Main, D.S. (August 2008) Processes of care desired by elderly patients with multimorbidities. *Family Practice*, **23** (4), 287–93.

Beasley, J. Hankey, T. Erickson, R. *et al.* (September 2004). How many problems do family physicians manage at each encounter? A WReN study. *Annals of Family Medicine*, **2** (5), 405–10.

Bower, P., Macdonald, W., Harkness, E. *et al.* (2011) Multimorbidity, service organization and clinical decision making in primary care: a qualitative study. *Family Practice*, **28** (5), 579–587.

Gijsen, R., Hoeymans, N., Schellevis, F.G., Ruwaard, D., Satariano, W.A. & van den Bos, G.A.M. (July 2001) Causes and consequences of comorbidity: a review. *Journal of Clinical Epidemiology*, **54** (7), 661–674.

Kerr, E.A., Heisler, M., Krein, S.L. *et al.* (December 2007) Beyond comorbidity counts: how do comorbidity type and severity influence diabetes patients' treatment priorities and self-management? *Journal of General Internal Medicine*, **22** (12), 1635–1640.

Noel, P.H., Frueh, C., Larme, A. & Pugh, J. (March 2005) Collaborative care needs and preferences of primary care patients with multimorbidity. *Health Expectations*, **8** (1), 54–63.

Parchman, M.L., Noel, P.H. & Lee, S. (2005) Primary care attributes, health care system hassles and chronic illness. *Medical Care*, **43** (11), 1123–1129.

Pham, H.H. Schrag, D. O'Malley, A.S. *et al.* (15 March 2007). Care patterns in Medicare and their implications for pay for performance. *New England Journal of Medicine*, **356** (11), 1130–9.

Shadmi, E., Boyd, C.M., Hsiao, C.J., Sylvia, M., Schuster, A.B. & Boult, C. (February 2006) Morbidity and older persons' perceptions of the quality of their primary care. *Journal of the American Geriatrics Society*, **54** (2), 330–334.

Tinetti, M.E. & Fried, T. (1 February 2004) The end of the disease era. *American Journal of Medicine*, **116** (3), 179–185.

Townsend, A., Hunt, K. & Wyke, S. (2003) Managing multiple morbidity in mid-life: a qualitative study of attitudes to drug use. *British Medical Journal*, **327**, 837.

Wolff, J.L., Starfield, B. & Anderson, G. (11 November 2002) Prevalence, expenditures, and complications of multiple chronic conditions in the elderly. *Archives of Internal Medicine*, **162** (20), 2269–2276.

CHAPTER 4

Effects of Multimorbidity on Healthcare Resource Use

Efrat Shadmi[1], Karen Kinder[2], and Jonathan P. Weiner[2]

[1] Faculty of Social Welfare and Health Sciences, Haifa University, Israel
[2] Department of Health Policy and Management, Bloomberg School of Public Health, The Johns Hopkins University, USA

OVERVIEW

- People with multimorbidity consume a disproportionately large share of healthcare resources
- Greater resource consumption is the result of not only greater need because of the accumulation of chronic diseases but also interactions and synergies between conditions present within individuals
- Multimorbidity measures have been shown to explain large variations (across populations/individual clinicians/healthcare organizations) in use of a range of healthcare resources – including inpatient services, specialized care, primary care and medications
- Multimorbidity has important implications for resource allocation within health systems as well as for care management programmes targeted at improving care and increasing care efficiency for high-risk multimorbid patients.

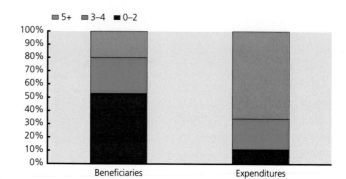

Figure 4.1 Distribution of US Medicare beneficiaries and expenditures by number of chronic conditions. Source: Data from Anderson and Horvath 2002. Derived from Medicare claims and beneficiary survey.

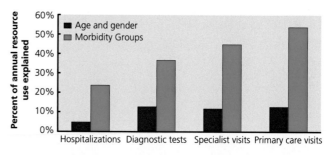

Figure 4.2 Explaining resource use with multimorbidity measures versus age and gender only. Morbidity groups: ADGs, Aggregate Diagnostic Groups (from the ACG system). Percentage represents the explained variance (R^2) from regression analysis. Source: Data from Shadmi et al. 2011.

Background

Context for understanding the impact of multimorbidity on healthcare resource use

People with multimorbidity consume a disproportionate amount of healthcare resources. Regardless of the way multimorbidity is defined (i.e. based on chronic condition counts, indices or measures of all types of conditions), higher levels of multimorbidity have consistently been shown to be associated with the largest share of resource consumption in numerous populations and settings around the globe (Lehnert, Heider, Leicht, *et al.*, 2011). The following examples, though based on data from individual countries, depict a picture representative of healthcare delivery worldwide. Figure 4.1 describes the characteristics and healthcare use for a cohort of older Americans (65+) in the government-sponsored Medicare programme. People with five or more chronic conditions constitute about a fifth of the Medicare population, yet consume two-thirds of all healthcare resources (Anderson, Horvath, 2002).

Figure 4.2 depicts the association between multimorbidity and primary care visits, specialist visits, performance of diagnostic tests and hospitalizations within Israel's Clalit Health Services,

which is an integrated delivery system. The analysis in this figure uses the Aggregate Diagnostic Groups (ADGs) of the of the Johns Hopkins Adjusted Clinical Groups® (ACG) system, discussed in Weiner (1991), which measures multimorbidity across all types of conditions (both acute and chronic) the patient may have. As shown in Figure 4.2, multimorbidity explains a much larger share of resource use for each of the four types of healthcare resources assessed compared with that of age and gender alone (Shadmi, Balicer, Kinder K, Abrams, Weiner, 2011) (See Box 4.1).

Causal pathways

While the phenomenon of high resource consumption in people with multimorbidity is well described, *how* multimorbidity results

ABC of Multimorbidity, First Edition.
Edited by Stewart W. Mercer, Chris Salisbury and Martin Fortin.
© 2014 John Wiley & Sons, Ltd. Published 2014 by John Wiley & Sons, Ltd.

Box 4.1 **How well can we predict which patients will make greatest use of healthcare resources?**

How exactly does multimorbidity lead to increased resource use? How can healthcare systems be designed to make the best and most efficient use of resources in the light of the growing prevalence of multimorbidity?

in excessive use of resources is less clear. Box 4.2 tells the story of how multimorbidity may result in high rates of resource use, using an example from the USA.

As depicted in Box 4.3, MM's healthcare resource use is determined by the highly professionalized fragmented nature of the healthcare system in the USA, with multiple sub-specialty experts and lack of coordinating mechanisms that can definitively ensure

Box 4.2 **Increased current and future resource use by levels of multimorbidity**

Using private insurance data for a two-year cohort of Americans under the age of 65, we describe (Figure 4.3) the group by multimorbidity percentile levels, as defined by the Johns Hopkins ACG multimorbidity index. This figure shows that the greater the multimorbidity, as measured by the index percentile levels (from 0 to 10% up to 95 to 99%), the greater the number of chronic conditions, total number of conditions and number of drug therapeutic classes used. We go on to assess the impact of this year's multimorbidity levels on future (year 2) resource use (Figure 4.4), showing a similar pattern. This 'predictive' type of analysis is critical for both reimbursement/budgeting (which usually uses past information to budget for future periods) and care management intervention designed to target and intervene individuals with the highest level of multimorbidity.

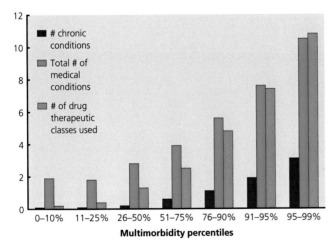

Figure 4.3 A cohort of insured under-65 Americans arrayed by multi-morbidity index percentile levels: Characteristics of each MM percentile group in year 1. Source: Johns Hopkins University. Unpublished data from a cohort of 904 007 persons below the age of 65 enrolled in private insurance plans for a two-year period. The multimorbidity index percentile ranking is based on the Johns Hopkins ACG predictive model, which calculates a morbidity burden risk score using morbidity markers derived from health insurance data for this cohort in 'year 1'.

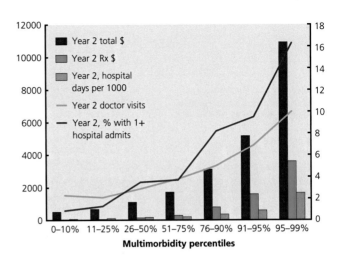

Figure 4.4 A cohort of insured under-65 Americans arrayed by multimorbidity index percentile levels: characteristics of each MM percentile group in year 2. Source: Johns Hopkins University. Unpublished data from a cohort of 904 007 persons below the age of 65 enrolled in private insurance plans for a two-year period. The multimorbidity index percentile ranking is based on the Johns Hopkins ACG predictive model, which calculates a morbidity burden risk score using morbidity markers derived from health insurance data for this cohort in 'year 1'.

Box 4.3 **Resource use by a 72-year-old man with multimorbidity**

MM is a 72-year-old man with diabetes, arthritis, ischaemic heart disease and chronic kidney disease. His care is provided for by several specialists, including an endocrinologist and neurologist for his complicated diabetes (recent peripheral neuropathy), a rheumatologist for his arthritis and a cardiologist for his ischaemic heart disease. Five months ago, MM was diagnosed with stage 2 chronic kidney disease and was asked to make an appointment with a nephrologist, which he has yet to schedule. MM also sees a dietician from the endocrinologists' clinic and a physiotherapist for his shoulder arthritis. MM sees his GP mainly when he runs out of his prescriptions, when he requires care for mild acute illnesses (such as laryngitis) or preventive services (such as flu vaccinations). During his last visit, his GP asked how his shoulder was doing. MM replied that it is much better now that he is on a new pain-relieving drug that his rheumatologist prescribed after there was no amelioration with the physiotherapy. The GP was surprised when MM told him that the rheumatologist was not aware of his new kidney disease diagnoses and that he had not yet seen the nephrologist. He recommended MM to go back to the rheumatologist and ask for a different line of treatment and to make the appointment with the nephrologist. He also ordered blood and urine laboratory tests to monitor his renal functions.

Ten days after the visit, the GP received a phone call from MM's wife who notified him that MM has just been discharged from the hospital (for which he was admitted because of high blood pressure and swelling of the legs and puffiness around his eyes), and that they were not sure if he should continue taking his 'old' medications (from before the hospitalization) or the newly hospital prescribed drugs.

the alignment of treatments and recommendations. In Figure 4.5, we offer a graphic depiction of how unnecessary resource use could occur for persons undergoing care for multiple conditions if there is sub-optimal coordination across separate episodes (especially in

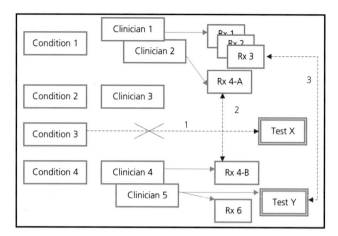

Figure 4.5 Examples of episode of care pathways where multimorbidity could impact resource use where coordination is sub-optimal.

specialist/consultant centric delivery systems). Without adequate coordination, omissions, duplications or contraindications could occur. These are represented by the three dotted lines in this figure, including omissions (line 1), duplications of treatment (line 2) or contraindications (as may occur in cases of incompatibility between treatments or between tests and treatments (line 3)).

Impact on inpatient and specialized care use

That multimorbidity is associated with high hospital use has been repeatedly shown in various healthcare settings and countries, using a wide range of approaches to quantifying multimorbidity and hospital services use, including total number of admissions, number of hospital days, readmissions, A&E (emergency department) use and outpatient specialty services. Having a combination of conditions creates challenges to care provision, as described earlier, and may result in inadequate control of one or more of the conditions, which, in turn, could put patients at higher risk for intensive healthcare resource use (most likely in the form of an in-patient hospitalization). As depicted in Box 4.3, people with multimorbidity rely on several types of specialists for their ongoing care. Exacerbations, due to the natural progression of the disease and/or to potential breakdowns in care, often result in hospitalization. This may lead to additional care for either follow-up or treatment of other conditions, which might have been affected by the care provided for the condition that instigated the hospitalization.

Impact on primary and preventive care use

People with multimorbidity are likely to be high users of primary and preventive care, for several reasons. First, patients often seek advice for undifferentiated symptoms (Salisbury, Johnson, Purdy, Valderas, Montgomery, 2011) (such as pain or shortness of breath) rather than a specific condition, thus consulting general practitioners (GPs) as the 'first contact' point of care. GPs are also often more accessible, both geographically and financially (with little or no copayments in most countries), factors that can positively affect the reliance on them as a major source of care for persons with multiple needs. GPs' role as providers of comprehensive care and

the ample opportunities created during patients' multiple visits can instigate higher use of preventive services, ranging from healthy life style recommendations to tertiary screening for the prevention of complications.

As coordinators, especially in delivery systems where the primary care doctor serves as a formal 'gateway', use of specialty care is contingent upon referral by the primary care clinician, thus higher use of specialty services can sometimes be paralleled by higher primary care visits. Lastly, primary care use also increases as a function of socio-demographic related needs, accruing within persons with multimorbidity as it is often the main source of care for persons of disadvantaged circumstances (Mercer, Guthrie, Furler, Watt, & Hart, 2012).

Impact on medication use and other services

While multiple medication use is common in people with multimorbidity, adherence to several Clinical Practice Guidelines (CPGs) (as indicated separately for each of the conditions) usually results in complicated treatment regimens involving a large number of medications (Figure 4.6). Increased medication use can have

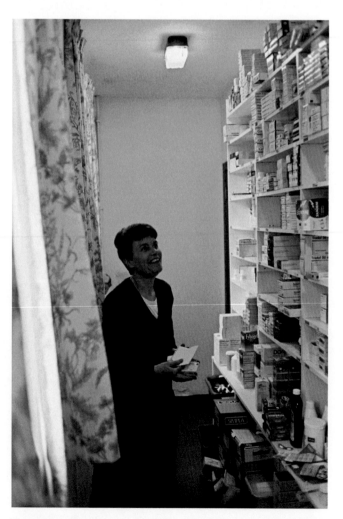

Figure 4.6 Multimorbidity is associated with polypharmacy and thus higher drug prescribing costs.

deleterious effects because of potential adverse effects and inter-actions between medications, resulting in increased use of other healthcare resources. In addition, drug costs can be quite sig-nificant, and depending on the insurance/delivery system, high out-of-pocket self-pay costs for the patient may also ensue. The relationship between multimorbidity burden and pharmacy costs is often nonlinear, as more expensive second-line drug regimens are often required because of interaction effects of multiple conditions.

Designing payment systems to take multimorbidity into consideration when compensating for resource use

Practices are facing pressures to deliver adequate care under cur-rent budget allocation formulae which fail to take into account the complex needs of multimorbid patients. Negotiations with fund-ing organizations have begun to raise this issue; however, further emphasis from practitioners is needed to ensure that the morbid-ity patterns of the patients' service are included in the allocation formula. Accounting for morbidity burden of patients and popu-lations in payment methodologies ensures that limited healthcare resources are directed to the persons (and the clinicians who serve them) who need these resources most.

Current methods of payment based on prior budgets or formu-las including only demographics or specific individual diseases may not adequately account for multimorbidity. Counting the number or type of individual chronic diseases is an advance over paying only by type of service (e.g. procedure codes) or demographic adjusted capitation, yet these methods only partially account for resource use (as shown in Figure 4.2). Furthermore, procedure-based payment may incorporate perverse incentives to deliver services, regardless of their appropriateness to the needs of the patient.

Multiple methodologies exist for measuring morbidity burden to account for patients' needs independent of measures of service use. However, before applying any method for clinician payment reim-bursement, a number of issues need to be considered and addressed:

- Adjusting payment or budgets for morbidities can be applied at various levels: regional, practice or individual clinician. The mor-bidity burden of clinicians' patient loads can be taken into account through weighted fee-for-service payments, morbidity-adjusted capitation formulae or offering a morbidity-based bonus to aug-ment clinicians' salaries.
- Accounting for morbidity can be applied either concurrently (based on the diagnoses presented during a current time period) or prospectively (predicting healthcare needs in a future year, based on diagnoses from a past period).
- As would be the case for any type of fixed budget or capitation payment (with or without morbidity adjustment), it is essential to define the services that will be included or 'carved out' from the payment methodology.
- It is also necessary to determine which practitioners the payment applies to (e.g. which type of doctor specialties, nurses or other allied professionals).

Challenges of including a morbidity measure in any budget allocation formula should be recognized. For instance, a patient may appear sicker when they have better access, thereby acquiring more diagnoses. In addition, variations in practices' morbidity bur-den may reflect clinician's code recording behaviour for diagnoses and not the variance in the morbidity of the patient population. Experience has shown that once practitioners understand that the accuracy and completeness of their recording of diagnoses impacts their remuneration, the quality of the records improves. In addition, establishing standards for electronic medical records facilitates comparative analyses.

Other special considerations when designing systems to ensure cost-effective resource use for patients with multimorbidity

There are many potential organizational changes that can be put in place when designing interventions that improve care quality and outcomes for persons with multimorbidity. In all cases, the issue of monitoring costs and seeking efficiency of resource use are paramount.

For example, it is essential to develop fair ways to assess per-formance (e.g. levels of hospital or pharmacy use). Incorporating a measure of multimorbidity in performance assessments helps to identify variation in health resource consumption that is *not* attributable to variation in illness among patients and/or popula-tions served. The causes of such variances could include systemic differences in the availability of services, patients' preferences or clinicians' practice behaviour, both positive (greater resource use might reflect more appropriate treatment) or negative (inappro-priate claiming of funds, waste, lack of competence). Once the clinicians who over- or under-utilize resources are identified, pro-grammes can be implemented to engage those clinicians in better understanding their behaviour as well as their patient population.

Recognition of multimorbidity is also relevant in identifying those multimorbid patients at high risk who could benefit from early interventions. To ensure effective and efficient use of limited resources, it is advantageous to apply existing methodologies to assist clinicians in this identification process. Such methodologies highlight the prevalence of disease clusters and the identification of trends within populations, and facilitate designing appropriate care intervention programmes which take into consideration the entire morbidity burden of multimorbid patients.

Conclusions

People with multimorbidity use a disproportionate amount of healthcare resources and in most nations worldwide, the percent-age of the population with multimorbidity is expected to increase significantly. These trends are happening at the same time when world economies are looking to constrain their ever-burgeoning outlay on societal healthcare expenditures. Current systems of care for people with multimorbidity are far from optimal, and there is wide variation on how resources are used. While there are tools for improving care efficiency to people with multimorbidity, these are not always applied. To ensure sustainability of health systems and meet the needs of multimorbid patients, it is essential to develop infrastructure and processes aimed towards optimal resource use as well as to work to expand our knowledge base through health services and clinical effectiveness research focused on how best to provide high-quality care that is also cost effective.

Further reading

Anderson G, Horvath J (2002). *Chronic conditions: Making the case for ongoing care*. Johns Hopkins University, Baltimore, MD. Retrieved from http://www.partnershipforsolutions.org/DMS/files/chronicbook2002.pdf

Lehnert, T., Heider, D., Leicht, H. *et al*. (2011) Review: Health care utilization and costs of elderly persons with multiple chronic conditions. *Medical Care Research and Review*, **68** (4), 387–420. doi:10.1177/1077558711399580

Mercer, S.W., Guthrie, B., Furler, J., Watt, G.C. & Hart, J.T. (2012) Multimorbidity and the inverse care law in primary care. *British Medical Journal*, **344**, e4152.

Salisbury, C., Johnson, L., Purdy, S., Valderas, J.M. & Montgomery, A.A. (2011) Epidemiology and impact of multimorbidity in primary care: A retrospective cohort study. *British Journal of General Practice*, **61** (582), e12–e21. doi:10.3399/bjgp11X548929

Shadmi, E., Balicer, R.D., Kinder, K., Abrams, C. & Weiner, J.P. (2011) Assessing socioeconomic health care utilization inequity in Israel: Impact of alternative approaches to morbidity adjustment. *BMC Public Health*, **11**, 609.

Weiner, JP, Starfield, BH, Steinwachs DM, Mumford LM (1991). Development and application of a population-oriented measure of ambulatory care case-mix. *Medical Care*, **29**(5), 452-472, www.acg.jhsph.edu

CHAPTER 5

Multimorbidity and the Primary Care Clinic

Stewart W. Mercer[1] and Chris Salisbury[2]

[1]General Practice and Primary Care, Institute of Health and Wellbeing, University of Glasgow, UK
[2]Centre for Academic Primary Care, NIHR School for Primary Care Research, School of Social and Community Medicine, University of Bristol, UK

OVERVIEW

- Primary care is largely organized around the needs of patients with single conditions, and thus patients with multimorbidity are like square pegs trying to be fitted into round holes
- Practices need to organize their care differently, putting the multimorbid patient at the centre of the system
- There is an urgent need to move from reactive to anticipatory care and from disease-centred approach to a holistic patient-centred approach
- This requires multiple changes at system, practitioner and patient levels
- Consultation length may need to be substantially increased for multimorbid patients combined with relational and informational continuities
- Self-management support needs to be enhanced both within consultations and by better links with community resources (community-facing primary care)
- In areas of high socio-economic deprivation, the problems facing multimorbid patients within primary care are exacerbated by the 'inverse care law', in which higher needs and demands result in poorer access, shorter consultations, lower patient enablement and increased GP stress.

Background

It will be clear by now from reading the previous chapters that although multimorbidity is the norm rather than the exception in patients with long-term conditions, healthcare systems remain largely configured around a single-disease model. The patient with multimorbidity can be compared to that of a square peg trying to be fitted into a series of round holes. The needs of multimorbid patients are often complex, involving not only several physical conditions but also psychological and social problems. Thus, the needs of patients with multimorbidity are likely to be best met by a holistic approach, based around generalist primary care.

So what is needed at practice level?

Since most health care received by multimorbid patients comes from primary care and general practitioners (GPs) in particular, the following discussion focuses mainly on the organization of general practice and primary care, although many of the issues are likely to be of similar importance in secondary care. Describing what is needed in the organization of care for patients with multimorbidity may be best illustrated by first thinking about what is not needed – yet is often what multimorbid patients encounter. What is not needed is rushed, fragmented episodic and reactive care delivered with a single-disease biomedical focus, with no coordination between providers and services and no regard for the burden imposed on the patient, nor the patients' views and priorities (see Box 5.1).

Box 5.1 **Example of reactive care of a multimorbid patient**

- Mr. D is a 58-year-old man who works night shift in the local supermarket staking shelves and suffers from COPD, hypertension, type 2 diabetes and back pain.
- He books an 'emergency' (same day) appointment to see Dr Y at his practice, a doctor he has never met before.
- The doctor is running 30 min late when he calls Mr. D into his consulting room.
- Mr. D explains that he has come about his cough and shortness of breath, and is finding it hard to cope with work because of this and his back pain. He is also finding it hard to sleep at home as high-rise flat he lives in is very noisy during the day.
- Dr Y only enquires about the cough, its duration, whether he is coughing up nasty coloured sputum or blood and his shortness of breath. He carries out a perfunctory examination of Mr. D's chest and tells him that he has a chest infection.
- He prescribes antibiotics and oral steroids, and a benzodiazepam to help him sleep. He gives him a sick note for two weeks saying 'unfit for work' but without any suggestions regarding a phased return to work or lighter duties.
- Dr Y is looking at his watch and ushers Mr. D out of his room, telling him to come back to see one of the doctors if things do not settle down.

ABC of Multimorbidity, First Edition.
Edited by Stewart W. Mercer, Chris Salisbury and Martin Fortin.
© 2014 John Wiley & Sons, Ltd. Published 2014 by John Wiley & Sons, Ltd.

What is needed of course is the complete reverse of this. Patient-centred care in its broadest sense is what is most needed in the care of multimorbid patients such as Mr. D, and the organization of care within the consultation, the practice and beyond needs to reflect such a focus. The issues critical to this include staff and patients' values and attitudes, the structure of consultations, consultation length, continuity and workload (on patients and healthcare staff). Practices can do much to organize the care they provide in a more patient-centred way, but many factors that influence this lie out with the remit of the GP or practice team. Policy and healthcare organization, on a macro-level, can greatly facilitate or hinder the possibility of optimal care for multimorbid patients and this is discussed in detail in Chapter 11.

How can this be achieved?

Moving from a reactive model of doctor (or nurse)-driven care to one that is anticipatory, inclusive, centred around the patient and his or her needs and priorities is no easy matter. Both financial and non-financial incentives may be important. Education and training of staff are also essential, as is the 'education' of patients as to what are realistic expectations, and honesty regarding what health care can and cannot achieve. Long-term conditions are by definition 'incurable' and patients should expect to receive holistic care that is responsive to their needs and priorities, but also need to recognize that doctors can only do so much, and they also have an important role as active participants in their own health and health care. However, we must caution against the development of a 'blame culture' and punitive actions against those who do not 'self-manage'. There are many barriers to effective self-management support for multimorbid patients within healthcare systems (Box 5.2)

Box 5.2 **What are the challenges of imbedding self-management support within consultations with patients with multimorbidity?**

- GPs worry that suggesting self-management may harm the doctor–patient relationship.
- GPs report a lack of time in the consultation to give self-management support.
- In deprived areas, GPs and practice nurses see the management of multimorbidity as an 'endless struggle' with self-management being low on the patients agenda.
- Community support (i.e. voluntary sector) is often singe disease focused.
- Patients in deprived areas need more help in accessing community information and support but GPs may not know what is available locally.

Identifying patients and recall systems

The first task in moving from reactive to anticipatory care for patients with multimorbidity requires that there are mechanisms in place within the clinic to accurately identify patients with multimorbidity. The effective management of these patients requires well-organized medical records, which increasingly depend on

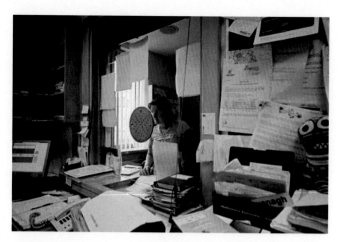

Figure 5.1 In many places, paper-based records remain the norm.

electronic health records leading to paperless or at least paper-light practices (unlike the example shown in Figure 5.1!).

Although this may seem a simple task in practices with electronic medical records, as pointed out in Chapter 7, the systematic recording of patients with multimorbidity within the electronic medical record often does not happen. In the UK, for example registers are recorded according to single diseases that are included in the Quality and Outcomes Framework (QOF). Searching the records to find which of these patients have multimorbidity is often difficult, especially when the conditions include those not currently included in the QOF targets. Thus, a primary task for practices, working in collaboration with IT providers, is to ensure that such searches can be done to identify target patients with multimorbidity and that recall systems are in place. This would ensure that it was then feasible to call specific patients for reviews, avoiding the common scenario of multimorbid patients being recalled to several single-disease clinics for review. An additional consideration is the burden of multimorbidity. The best way to measure and document multimorbidity burden routinely in clinical IT systems is not clear, but a simple count of the number of chronic conditions per patient correlates well with other validated measures of multimorbidity burden (see Figure 5.2). The best method of predicting health service utilization is also unclear but again, a simple count may be as predictive as other methods at least for certain outcomes (Table 5.1).

Informational and relational continuity

The second task in developing a patient-centred practice for multimorbidity is to have a system in place that supports continuity of care. Informational continuity, in which key information about a patient is held within the clinical record, so that different doctors within the practice can access this information, is of course a basic pre-requisite of any attempt at improving continuity. However, for many patients with multimorbidity, relational continuity is important to both patient and doctor. For the patient, seeing the same doctor at each visit or most visits decreases the need to repeat their story and enhances trust and the development of a therapeutic relationship. For the doctor, it is also important clinically and interpersonally, and can save time as old ground does not need to

Table 5.1 Relationship between different measures of multimorbidity burden and health service utilization.

	Number of GP clinic visits	Number of prescribed drugs	Number of blood tests	Number of hospital out-patient visits	Number of A + E (Accident and Emergency) visits	Number of unplanned hospital admissions
Multimorbidity count	0.56***	0.64***	0.59***	0.32**	0.28**	0.28**
CIRS	0.63***	0.71***	0.61***	0.28**	0.24*	0.32**
Charlson	0.41***	0.48***	0.25**	0.32**	0.24*	0.22*
ACG	0.68***	0.68***	0.48***	0.39***	0.38***	0.34***

Unpublished data from Stewart W. Mercer, on 106 general practice patients in Scotland. Results show Spearman's correlation coefficients (rho). *$P < 0.05$, **$P < 0.01$ and ***$P < 0.001$.

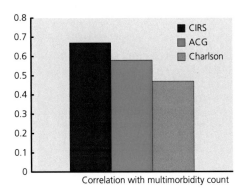

Figure 5.2 Relationship between number of chronic conditions and measures of burden. Unpublished data from Stewart W. Mercer on 200 primary care patients with multimorbidity in Scotland. Correlations between total multimorbidity count and all three measures of burden were significant ($P < 0.001$).

be gone over at each meeting. With changes in practice, such as a greater emphasis on rapid access to care and more GPs and health-care staff working part-time, relational continuity can be hard to achieve. However, for multimorbid patients having a lead GP (and in secondary care a lead specialist) that the patient sees most of the time, with one or two other GPs that they see when the lead GP is not available, would be an improvement. This would then require that the GPs responsible for the care of that patient were kept well informed about decisions made (i.e. communication between GPs within the practice would be required) and can act as an overall coordinator of care.

Healthcare systems can promote or hinder continuity of care (Boxes 5.3 and 5.4).

Box 5.3 **Improving continuity of care for patients with multiple conditions in general practice (data from Hill and Freeman 2011).**

- Ensure that patients with multimorbidity understand that doctors find it easier to provide good care for patients they know well. This is especially important for people from socio-economically deprived populations who have the greatest burden of illness, the greatest need for continuity of care and the lowest ability to navigate administrative barriers which may get in the way of them seeing a regular doctor.
- Change receptionists' behaviour and the prompts on booking systems so that the patient's 'own doctor' becomes the default option.

- Organize large practices into small teams of two or three doctors who see each other's patients when one is away. Ensure that patients know about these arrangements.
- Identify patients with particularly complex problems who should only be seen by a restricted number of doctors. Adjust the appointment system so that they cannot be booked into other doctors. Explain this to the patients, this means they may have to wait longer for an appointment but they will get better care for their complex problems.
- Develop better questions on continuity of care in patient surveys and make sure they are included in patient assessments of care. Where countries have arrangements for regular appraisal of doctors or periodic revalidation or recertification, include questions on how a doctor's practice is organized to provide continuity of care for people with complex problems.

Box 5.4

What are the 'ingredients' of good consultations in multimorbidity from the patients perspective and from the doctors?
How might the profile of the practice population (e.g. a practice in a high deprivation area) influence the consultation?
What are the likely solutions to improving care for multimorbid patients within primary care?

Time

Clinics and practices are usually very busy places, and time is at a premium. In the UK, general practices usually run on a 10-min booked appointment time, irrespective of the patient and the reason for consulting. For multimorbid patients consulting about complex issues, this is often inadequate, especially when the medical problems are compounded by social problems as is often the case in areas of high deprivation. In such situations, either the doctor strictly time limits the consultations to avoid running late, and in so doing ignores or minimizes some of the multimorbid patient's concerns and needs, or the doctor runs late, disrupting the clinic and increasing doctor stress.

Continuity of care may help time management. Multimorbid patients consult more frequently than other patients and if continuity of care is good, then both patient and doctor can discuss issues raised in the consultation in the context of serial encounters, knowledge about the problems and a long-term relationship.

However, there is also a strong case for more time for targeted patients with multimorbidity. Not all multimorbid patients will need longer consultations at every visit. However, some may benefit from longer encounters. For example, patients with several long-term physical conditions may benefit from regular structured longer review (perhaps every six months) to assess the patient holistically, and to review important issues such as mental health, functional ability and polypharmacy. Other patients may require a more frequent 'stepping up' of care, when problems have increased and are becoming unmanageable for the patient (such as following a new diagnosis and additional treatment regimen). In such circumstances, care may need to be intensified in a series of longer consultations focused on the patient's priorities and needs, until the patient and the situation stabilize. Building flexibility into the routine appointment systems of busy clinics is not an easy task, and each practice needs to develop a system that best suits the needs of the patient population they serve. There has been limited research on the best ways to implement longer consultations and the benefit of them. However, in one study in an area of high deprivation, simply adding extra time slots within booked surgeries, so that if a patient presented with complex needs extra time could be allocated there and then, led to improvements in patient enablement and reductions in GP stress (Mercer et al. 2007).

Putting the 'care' into health care

As has been repeatedly emphasized in this book, multimorbidity is not simply about a combination of long-term conditions that need to be managed effectively as individual conditions, but is about the wide-ranging effects it has on the individual, their family and indeed society as a whole. As such, it is therefore essential that patients receive comprehensive care that takes a holistic approach to understanding the problems faced by patients. Holistic care cannot be achieved by a mechanistic tick-box approach. Holistic care requires human care, and practitioners need to be perceived by their patients as empathic. Without this basic ingredient, little will be achieved. Empathy is a basic pre-requisite for patient enablement (Mercer et al. 2012a). Patients with multimorbidity value empathy in their healthcare encounters (see Figure 5.3) and so empathy needs to be embraced, encouraged and if necessary taught to healthcare practitioners (Bikker et al. 2012).

However, empathy alone is insufficient in the management of multimorbid patients. Practitioners also need to be skilled generalists, so that they can recognize and respond to a variety of clinical situations. GPs are of course well placed to serve this role, as long as they receive sufficient training and support. Hospital generalists are also very important though, and the demise of the generalist physician in the wake of increasing specialism and sub-specialism is clearly at odds with the needs of many patients with multimorbidity.

Care planning and self-management

A key tenet of the chronic care model (Chapter 11) is the need to support patients with long-term conditions to manage their own conditions. However, support for self-management is often limited in primary care, and patients with multimorbidity face particular

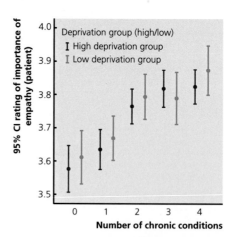

Figure 5.3 Multimorbid patients value empathy in the GP consultation. Unpublished data from Mercer et al. (2012a) showing the effect of increasing multimorbidity on patients' views on the importance of GP empathy within the clinical encounter. Study of over 3000 patients, approximately half living in areas of high socio-economic deprivation (poor areas) and another half living in areas of low socio-economic deprivation (richer areas).

problems with self-management, which are described in more depth in Chapters 3 and 9.

Multimorbid patients need to have their care carefully planned whenever possible, and many countries are introducing care plans to support this. These are usually written records of a plan based on agreed priorities, goals and actions, with planned follow-up and review. Care plans fit well with the chronic care model (see Chapter 11), and must to be tailored to the patients' needs and priorities. Care planning in multimorbidity may require considerable time and skill, given the common complexity of needs, and factors to consider. Care plans are not just about what the patient can do to help themselves (e.g. goal setting in self-management) but also about planning future healthcare needs. For example, the transition from primary care to secondary care is often unplanned and un-coordinated, prompted perhaps by an acute illness. Once in hospital, the coordination with primary care and social services to enable a timely discharge is also often poorly organized. By working more closely, primary care and secondary care could do much more to make the transition from primary care to secondary care (and back) seamless and efficient.

The importance of practice context

Multimorbidity shows a marked 'social gradient', being more common in patients of lower socio-economic status (Figure 5.4; see also Chapter 2). The complexity of consultations is greatest when multimorbidity involves both physical and mental health conditions, as is commonly the case (see Chapter 5). Mental health problems are much more common in deprived areas, and thus the relationship between multimorbidity of physical conditions and mental health conditions is socially patterned, with a step-wise increase in mental illness associated with multimorbidity as deprivation rises. This raises important issues for practices serving areas of concentrated deprivation, where an inverse care law usually operates (Table 5.2). In such practices, patients with such complex

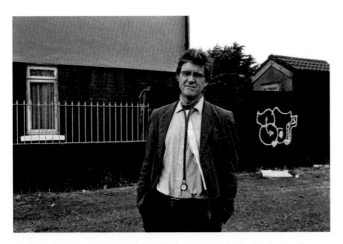

Figure 5.4 GPs working in areas of high socio-economic deprivation face many challenges, not least of which is the continuing existence of the inverse care law.

Table 5.2 How the inverse care law affects general practice in deprived areas.

Higher patient demand
More multimorbidity
More mental illness
More social problems
More complex needs
More problems to discuss
Poorer access to GP
Shorter consultations
Less patient enablement
Higher GP stress
Poorer outcomes

needs feel less enabled by consultations with their GPs than similar patients in more affluent areas, and their GPs feel more stressed (Mercer and Watt 2007). Therefore, the need for greater continuity of care and for more time in consultations is particularly important in deprived areas. Doctors working in deprived areas face a 'triple-whammy' of a generally higher consultation rate, a higher prevalence of multimorbidity and more challenging consultations complicated by interactions between social, mental and physical problems. In these circumstances, doctors are likely to need smaller caseloads and greater resources in order to provide optimal care.

Conclusions

Multimorbid patients have complex needs that need to be addressed in the clinical encounter, and practices need to organize their care so that the multimorbid patient is at the centre of the system not at the periphery. A holistic patient-centred approach is required at system, practitioner and patient levels.

Sufficient time in the consultation and comprehensive continuity of care are essential to deal with the complex acute and chronic medical problems, to build trust and to help empower patients. Care plans that reflect the patients' priorities and goals, including realistic and achievable self-management strategies, are an important tool in recording and reflecting on achievements over time and when used wisely can strengthen the motivation of both patient and practitioner.

Further reading

Bikker, A.P., Mercer, S.W. & Cotton, P. (2012) Connecting, Assessing, Responding and Empowering (CARE): a universal approach to person-centred, empathic healthcare encounters. *Education in Primary Care*, **23** (6), 454–457.

Hill, A.P. & Freeman, G.K. (2011) *Promoting Continuity of Care in General Practice*. Royal College of General Practitioners, London.

Jani, B.D., Blane, D.N. & Mercer, S.W. (2012) The role of empathy in therapy and the physician-patient relationship. *Research in Complementary Medicine*, **19** (5), 2–2. doi:10.1159/000342998

Mercer, S.W. & Watt, G.M.C. (2007) The inverse care law: clinical primary care encounters in deprived and affluent areas of Scotland. *Annals of Family Medicine*, **5**, 503–510.

Mercer, S.W., Jani, B., Wong, S.Y. & Watt, G.C.M. (2012a) Patient enablement requires physician empathy: a cross-sectional study of general practice consultations in areas of high and low socioeconomic deprivation in Scotland. *BMC Family Practice*, **13**, 6.

Mercer SW, Guthrie B, Furler J, Watt GCM, Hart JT. Multimorbidity and the inverse care law in primary care. *British Medical Journal* 2012b, **344**:e4152. doi: 10.1136/bmj.e4152

Mercer, S.W., Fitzpatrick, B., Gourlay, G., Vojt, G., McConnachie, A. & Watt, G.C.M. (2007) More time for complex consultations in a high deprivation practice is associated with increased patient enablement. *British Journal of General Practice*, **57**, 960–966.

CHAPTER 6

Multimorbidity and Patient-Centred Care

Moira Stewart[1] *and Martin Fortin*[2]

[1]Centre for Studies in Family Medicine, Western University, Schulich School of Medicine and Dentistry, Western Centre for Public Health and Family Medicine, Canada
[2]Family Medicine Department, Université de Sherbrooke, Academic Research Director, Centre de Santé et de Services Sociaux de Chicoutimi, Canada

OVERVIEW

- Patient-centredness was born from the need to understand the patient's experience and to integrate this experience into care
- A patient-centred approach to consultations avoids several common pitfalls encountered with multimorbid patients
- A patient-centred approach includes four components: exploring the diseases and the patients' illness experience; understanding the whole person in context; finding common ground and enhancing the patient–practitioner relationship
- Research has shown that patient-centred consultations positively affect outcomes.

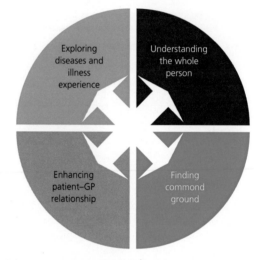

Figure 6.1 Four components of patient-centred GP consultations.

Introduction

Throughout the history of medicine two approaches have been used: a basic biomedical approach seeking answers to single pathologies, and a more Hippocratic approach seeking to place the pathology into a context that includes the patient's experience and environment. Current manifestations of these broad approaches are evidence-based medicine-producing key guidelines of the quality of care for each chronic condition, and person-based medicine seeking to integrate the patient's experience and context into care. A healthcare practitioner wishing to provide the best care for his or her patients with multimorbidity may need to find a way of incorporating or integrating these two broad approaches. The patient-centred clinical method offers such an integrated framework.

Box 6.1

What are the four principal components of the patient-centred consultation?
What are the outcomes that have shown to be positively affected by patient-centred care?
What are the common pitfalls that can be avoided with multimorbidity patients by using a patient-centred approach?

Patient centredness is especially relevant to the care of patients with multimorbidity as the diseases and the illness experience form an interwoven pattern that is often impossible to disentangle and that should be dealt with as a whole. This chapter introduces the components of patient-centred care as a framework for the medical consultation adapted to the care of patients with multimorbidity.

Although several models of patient-centredness have been suggested, we present here the essential components as a guide to help organize the consultation of the general practitioner (GP) with multimorbid patients. However, these components are applicable to most if not all healthcare practitioners' consultations. The consultation should focus on four essential components depicted in Figure 6.1: exploring the diseases and the patient's illness experience including expectations; understanding the whole person in context; finding common ground including agreeing on competing priorities and enhancing the patient–GP relationship. The components are guides and, with each patient, they combine in an interconnected manner. Over time, a practitioner will weave back and forth among the four components in providing continuity of care.

Multimorbidity contributes to the particular context of a consultation because it evolves over time as old conditions may worsen or become salient and new conditions are added. Multimorbidity is chronic but unlikely to be stable. Patients are thus facing an

ABC of Multimorbidity, First Edition.
Edited by Stewart W. Mercer, Chris Salisbury and Martin Fortin.
© 2014 John Wiley & Sons, Ltd. Published 2014 by John Wiley & Sons, Ltd.

increasingly complex experience over time, and it is therefore very important that the GP be patient-centred and adapt to this evolving challenge.

This patient-centred approach to the consultation avoids several common pitfalls encountered with multimorbid patients. It avoids too much attention on one disease at a time, a problem especially when some prevalent conditions require common management strategies, such as lifestyle modification. In addition, it avoids unnecessary subsequent recurring visits of patients, thus reducing healthcare costs. Also, it stresses the continuity of the relationship with the patient over many consultations, thereby helping to prevent feelings of failure and, even, abandonment, in patients when the conditions worsen. All in all, a focus on the person is more likely to meet patients' needs (Box 6.1).

Justification for a patient-centred approach

The main justification for a patient-centred approach is that it is the right approach to take – the moral imperative. As well, there are additional justifications. Firstly, patients expect consultations that include the four components listed earlier. Secondly, multimorbidity is so prevalent that an approach that addresses each chronic problem as separate and distinct makes no sense practically or conceptually. Akin to the second argument is the fact that the majority of GP patients have different sorts of illness experiences such as feelings, ideas about what is wrong, expectations of their health care, effects on their daily function and relevant contextual issues regarding family or work. Figure 6.2 demonstrates the magnitude of these relevant illness issues, driving home the notion that flexibility and a patient-oriented approach are necessary. Thirdly, research has shown that patient-centred consultations positively affect a list of important outcomes, desired by practitioners, patients and the healthcare system (see Box 6.2 for the list of outcomes).

First component: exploring diseases and the illness experience

One of the key problems in working with patients with long-term conditions is the somewhat false sense of security, because the

> **Box 6.2 Outcomes affected by patient-centred care**
>
> - Patients are more satisfied
> - Patients report more positive experiences of their health care
> - Patients are more likely to adhere to the treatment plan
> - Patients report improved symptoms
> - Patients report decreased anxiety
> - Patients' functional status improves
> - Utilization and costs decrease

clinician already knows the diagnoses. The clinician might therefore assume too much. However, the patient will experience a new reality with each GP consultation: different patient feelings which may impede treatment/management; different ideas and beliefs about the conditions and the preferred treatment plan; different expectations of the GP and the primary healthcare team; and different levels of function that may offer clues to exacerbation or to barriers to the management plan. Patient's illness experience varies overtime as new elements occur; feelings may evolve, expectations may change based on new facts, new symptoms or new limitations. Multimorbidity can causes confusion for the patient as the same symptoms may indeed originate from different conditions and need to be dealt with differently. This confusion is part of the illness experience and should be understood by the GP. Therefore, the first task of the consultation is to explore and re-explore these dimensions of the patient's illness experience and incorporate them, in a flexible manner, into the ongoing treatment/management plan (see Box 6.3 for a case example).

> **Box 6.3**
>
> Rex is 58 years old, eight months post-triple artery bypass surgery, with hypertension and celiac disease as well. He is dieting and exercising and his GP monitors these behaviours carefully. But Rex's sadness when discussing winter activities with his family took the GP by surprise. 'So many things have been taken away from me.' The opportunity for the GP is to follow this opening with a discussion of Rex's feelings and fears. The danger of dismissing this opening is that a true depression could be missed and also that unexpressed non-depressive feelings could overwhelm Rex and impede his adjustment and healing.

Second component: understanding the whole person in context

People who are diagnosed with multiple long-term conditions are often shocked or saddened that their bodies have let them down. This impact varies among different people and is influenced by the person's life history to date, their stage of life as well as their personality. For example, a rebellious adolescent with new and multiple long-term conditions is quite different from a retired senior who has become more resilient. Furthermore, the patients' context (family, school or employment, social support) needs to be

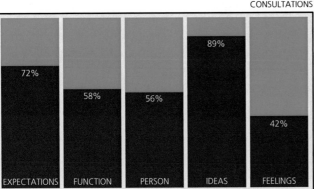

311 GP
CONSULTATIONS

Figure 6.2 Patient issues expressed during consultations with their GP.

explored and its positive influence maximized. Finally, the patient's cultural, community and neighbourhood environment may impact on the conditions or the evolving management plans (see Box 6.4 for a case example).

Box 6.4

John is 75, hemiplegic, with diabetes, hypertension and arthritis; his 65-year-old wife, Susan, has osteoporosis, asthma and a mild heart condition, and is John's main caregiver at home. Their GP and other primary care professionals must constantly take into account his family, his home and community support, in order to adequately care for John and Susan. 'I do not want John to go to a nursing home (long-term care).' Short-term relief was offered and the balance was restored but caring for the whole person in context will be the ongoing challenge for John and Susan's GP.

Third component: finding common ground

It is often difficult for practitioners to understand why many patients do not follow the suggested management plan. It may be because the patient has different priorities than the doctor. It may even be because the patient does not agree with the seriousness of the symptoms exhibited or may have other explanations for the symptoms, as in the example in Box 6.5. In order to sort out such potential disagreements, the doctor can engage in a discussion with the patient about the nature and priority of the multiple long-term conditions as well as the goals of management and what role the patient is able to play in meeting these agreed-upon goals.

Box 6.5 **Agreement on the problems**

A survivor of breast cancer diagnosed three years ago, Cynthia, 59, dismisses her back pain. Her GP believes it might be due to metastases. She believes it is osteoporosis and her osteoarthritis that have worsened. Therefore, she is not interested in having her back pain investigated, as she finds this irrelevant. Her GP has to deal with the competing interpretations of the complex symptoms as they may impede speedy diagnosis and progress toward an agreed-upon plan of action by Cynthia and her GP.

As seen in the earlier section, doctors have to consider contextual factors not only to understand the patient but also to ensure that the actions required from the patient will end-up being feasible with the least interference with their life and activities. Multimorbidity brings additional complexity by multiplying the numbers of recommendations that could apply. The doctor needs to take this into consideration and avoid discouraging the patient with too complex care plan. Compromises may be required to account for the patient's context and sometimes progressive implementation of recommendations might represent a good alternative as seen in Box 6.6.

Box 6.6

James is 55, presenting hypertension, obesity and osteoarthritis. He is a businessman with a busy schedule who travels a lot. Newly diagnosed with diabetes, James is eligible for a referral to a diabetic programme offered at the local health facility over a one-week period. James does not wish to be referred to this programme, as it does not fit into his busy schedule. His GP offers that James meet with a nurse to adapt an education programme taking into account the multiple long-term conditions over the next six or eight months and to start taking medication. A follow-up with the GP is planned. James is happy with this compromise.

Fourth component: enhancing the patient–practitioner relationship

Being a patient with multimorbidity is disheartening, as it can be profoundly discouraging. Supporting the patient in this difficult and ongoing journey takes empathy ('This is just so hard'), consistency ('I am going to stay with you through this') and hope ('Together we will get through this"). Over time, patients learn to trust the support offered by the GP and others and to trust their own ability to cope with their conditions. In the context of multimorbidity, a good relationship with the GP is essential as the patient's experience with health care is likely to be chaotic at some point. Patients have to deal with several medical specialists, healthcare professionals and staff. They also have to navigate in a healthcare system that becomes more complex as the complexity of their own situation increases. In this context, the ongoing relationship with a GP is essential as he or she is often the only provider who is consistently involved and can understand and support them in this journey (Figure 6.3). One cannot underestimate the importance of this role (see Box 6.7 for a case example).

We have seen in this chapter that the patient-centred approach is particularly important when multiple long-term conditions are present. The art of being a good healthcare practitioner is to be able to combine medical science with knowledge of patients as people, their experiences, their values and their beliefs within their particular context, with an ongoing and positive relationship.

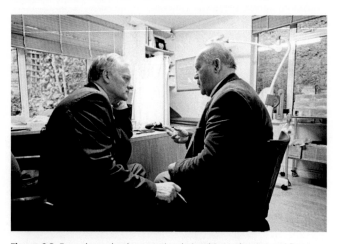

Figure 6.3 Empathy and a therapeutic relationship are key in providing patient-centred care to patients with multimorbidity.

Box 6.7

Helen, 68, has had a long story of use of the healthcare system. Diabetic since the age of 40, she underwent a liver transplant five years ago for non-alcoholic cirrhosis. Most recently, she underwent an aortic valve replacement that was complicated by a pulmonary embolism. Being also asthmatic, she feels very worried and frightened when she experiences shortness of breath. Being treated by several medical specialists in different facilities, she is very upset by the prescriptions she receives from all of them and needs to be reassured that they are required. She comes to her GP's office every three months to discuss her experience with the healthcare system and to verify if the treatments she is receiving are suitable. The reason she comes is because she trusts the GP who has been there for her for the last 25 years and she needs his counsel, otherwise she could not cope.

Further Reading

Bikker, A.P., Mercer, S.W. & Cotton, P. (November 2012) Connecting, Assessing, Responding and Empowering (CARE): a universal approach to person-centred, empathic healthcare encounters. *Education for Primary Care*, **23** (6), 454–457.

Hudon, C., Fortin, M., Haggerty, J., Loignon, C., Lambert, M. & Poitras, M.-E. (2012) Patient-centered care in chronic disease management: a thematic analysis of the literature in family medicine. *Patient Education and Counseling*, **88**, 170–176.

Stewart, M.A., Belle Brown, J.B., Weston, W.W., McWhinney, I.R., McWilliam, C.L. & Freeman, T.R. (2003) *Patient-Centered Medicine: Transforming the Clinical Method*, 2nd edn. Radcliffe Medical Press Ltd, Oxford.

CHAPTER 7

Multimorbidity and the Healthcare Electronic Medical Record

Amanda L. Terry[1] and Sonny Cejic[2,3]

[1]Centre for Studies in Family Medicine, Department of Family Medicine and Department of Epidemiology & Biostatistics, Schulich School of Medicine & Dentistry, The University of Western Ontario, Canada
[2]Department of Family Medicine, Schulich School of Medicine & Dentistry, The University of Western Ontario, Canada
[3]Byron Family Medical Centre, Canada

OVERVIEW

- Current electronic medical record (EMR) systems are limited in their capacity to support the care of patients with multimorbidity
- EMRs need to be used comprehensively and integrated fully into healthcare practice to maximize their usefulness
- Information should be entered into EMRs in a way that it supports comprehensive use – this is the foundation for allowing practitioners to begin to harness the power of the EMR
- Computer-based technology, in the form of advanced EMRs, is necessary to support the complexity of care required by patients with multimorbidity.

The electronic medical record (EMR) is a specialized kind of computer software that is used by health care practitioners to support the care of their patients. Current EMR systems are generally structured to reflect a single-disease orientation and are used in this way by primary healthcare practitioners. This is a significant limitation as some of the functions of current EMRs, for example, algorithms to identify patients with specific conditions, are too simplistic to use with patients who have multimorbidity. However, this is the current reality of EMR use in primary health care. Therefore, this chapter focuses on the use of EMRs in the care of patients with multimorbidity from two perspectives: (1) maximizing the use of current EMRs, and (2) how future EMRs could better support the care of these patients.

How can existing EMR technology be best used for the care of patients with multimorbidity?

To best use the current EMRs to support the care of patients with multimorbidity, it is important to pay attention to five key tasks as follows (Terry *et al.* 2012).

1 Use the EMR comprehensively in day-to-day practice
   This means using all of the parts of the software program that are available and clinically relevant to the fullest extent possible.

Currently, many practitioners do not use their EMRs fully (Figure 7.1).

To achieve more comprehensive use, primary healthcare practitioners should: (1) engage in targeted software training, (2) have a 'super-user' or coach, someone who can help in the use of the EMR software, (3) have a system whereby feedback reports are created; for example, immunizations completed for all patients, on a regular basis. This allows the practitioner to both reflect on the quality of the information being entered and to develop skills in retrieving information from the EMR.

2 Organize the practice to support the tasks that emerge from EMR use
   Organization involves attending to change the management processes, including workflows and the re-organization of human resources. For example, if reminders are generated within the EMR for follow-ups in patient care, how can these tasks be handled by the practice? What resources need to be in place to support this work?

3 Attend to and coordinate data entry practices
   Attend to data entry practices and coordinate these with the practices of the larger primary healthcare team (Ryan *et al.* 2011). For example, the recording of information using structured data (using systems such as the International Classification of Primary Care) *versus* information recorded in an unstructured or narrative manner (Figure 7.2).
   Periodic chart audits should be conducted to assess the quality of data that is recorded.

4 Organize patient summaries
   Organize patient summaries in the problem list so that it immediately becomes apparent that the patient has multimorbidity when the chart is opened. It is also important to understand how the coding of this list in the practitioner's particular EMR works – is the coding specific enough that the nature of the multimorbidity is clear? As an additional step, review patient summaries and problem lists regularly.

5 Include the EMR in the encounter
   Finally, how the EMR is used in the encounter with the patient, particularly in terms of how the information is gathered from the patient, can affect the quality of the information in the EMR. For this reason, the practitioner needs to attend to the interaction of themselves with the patient and the EMR during the encounter. There are three main things to keep in mind: (1) the structure

ABC of Multimorbidity, First Edition.
Edited by Stewart W. Mercer, Chris Salisbury and Martin Fortin.
© 2014 John Wiley & Sons, Ltd. Published 2014 by John Wiley & Sons, Ltd.

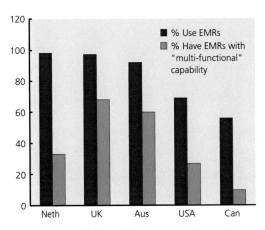

Figure 7.1 Primary care physician EMR use – comparison in five countries. Data from Schoen *et al*. 2012.

Level of Structure	Type of Data	Examples
Unstructured Data	Scanned documents	Historical paper records
		Lab results
		Consultation letters
		Images
	Narrative fields	Clinical notes
	Free-format fields No conventions	Multiple ways of entering condition (e.g. -diabetes, DM, diabetic)
	Free format fields Conventions	Consistent entry for condition e.g. 'diabetes'not DM or diabetic
	Structured fields	Pick lists
		Radio on/off buttons
Structured Data		Date formatted fields
DM - diabetes mellitus, EMR - electronic medical record		

Figure 7.2 Taxonomy of EMR data structure. Source: Ryan *et al*. (2011). Reproduced by permission from College of Family Physicians of Canada.

of the space used for the interview, (2) the attentiveness of the practitioner to the computer and the patient and (3) the way the patient interacts with the computer (Figures 7.3 and 7.4).

How could future EMRs better support the care of patients with multimorbidity?

There are three key areas within which EMRs and accompanying information technology could evolve to better support the care of patients with multimorbidity: (1) improved primary healthcare practitioner and patient access to the EMR, (2) enhanced EMR capacity to support team-based care and information needs and (3) advanced EMR functioning to facilitate patient care.

Improved access to the EMR

Improvements in the access to the EMR are needed to facilitate the use of this technology by practitioners and patients. Practitioners need to be able to access the EMR remotely during out-of-office activities or in-home patient visits using multiple methods; for example, via hand-held devices or secure websites.

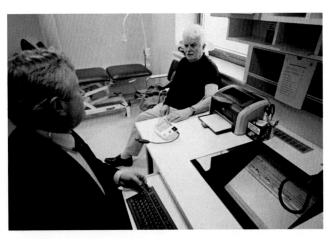

Figure 7.3 Modern IT systems are essential for high-quality care of multimorbid patients, but the way computers are used within the consultation is also important.

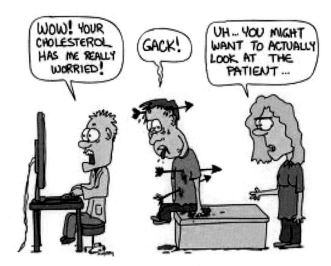

Figure 7.4 In the treatment room, patients cannot compete with a computer. Source: http://www.drmussey.com/ (as appeared in The Free Lance Star May 27, 2011). Reproduced with permission from Dr Steven Mussey.

Patients need to be able to view their medical records, enter data into the EMR, confirm information that is present and to engage in self-monitoring activities potentially through individualized access to specific areas of the EMR. One way patient data may be entered in the EMR is through home clinical measurement devices; for example, an electronic blood pressure cuff could measure values and send the information securely to the practitioner's EMR (Figure 7.5). Finally, primary healthcare practitioners need to be able to communicate directly with the patients using electronic means such as secure emailing, texting and messaging within the patient-accessed areas of the EMR.

Enhanced EMR capacity to support team-based care and information needs

Team-based care is a key aspect of providing excellent primary health care for patients who have multimorbidity; future EMRs need to be configured to support this type of care. In addition,

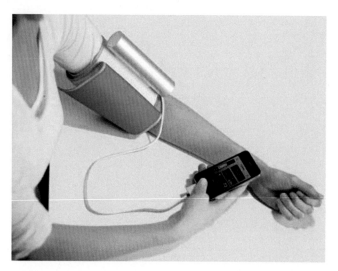

Figure 7.5 Example of a blood pressure cuff (Withings Smart Blood Pressure Monitor).

EMRs need to support the information needs of practitioners in the care of patients with multimorbidity. To achieve these goals, several developments are required. 'User-friendly' EMRs need to be designed that facilitate team-based care, with features such as a shared medical problem-coding system among practitioners, and support for the data entry and care-provision needs of different practitioners. Electronic communication and appropriate electronic exchange of information among practitioners are also necessary to support team-based care. Ease of information entry is important; for example, having the computer-coding information in the background while the practitioner is caring for the patient in the encounter. To facilitate care, key elements in the problem list and patient history should be tailored to the individual patient's characteristics and should be immediately available when the practitioner opens the patient's chart. In addition, the EMR needs to present summaries of patient information to the practitioner; for example, flagging out-of-range clinical values for that individual.

Advanced EMR functions

Care of patients with multimorbidities also requires a shift in clinical thinking – away from a focus on individual conditions to that of the complex reality of patients with multiple and co-occurring conditions. EMRs need to be designed to mirror this reality. An 'active EMR' with advanced functions could be developed to support the care of patients with multimorbidity, where information specific to the individual patient would be continually sought, analyzed and summarized by the computer. For example, the EMR could scan the literature for recent changes in medical evidence and present lists of patients to the practitioner who are affected by these changes. This could facilitate follow-up activities by the practitioner; for example, sending a secure email to a patient who needs a medication change. In addition, the EMR could calculate probabilities of potential diagnoses of multimorbidity and display them to the practitioner when the patient is present. This would be based on information entered in the EMR; for example, test results, history, symptoms and diagnoses from specialists.

New algorithms to warn a practitioner of concerning interactions could be developed as part of this kind of EMR. Similar to the medication-to-medication interaction function, medication-to-disease interaction checks for patients with multiple conditions and medications could be implemented. For example, an alert stating the consequences of prescribing a beta-blocker medication in a patient with asthma or sick-sinus syndrome. Within the patient encounter, the EMR could (1) provide ideal decision support, by seeking information from best practice sources and summarizing the evidence for individual patients with multimorbidity to support the development of the care plan, (2) assist the practitioner by producing 'care plan scenarios' based on individual patients with specific clusters of conditions, (3) calculate the convergence and divergence among multiple clinical practice guidelines and (4) present options for the optimal management of patients with multimorbidity.

A recent commentary (Dawes 2010) suggests that 'risk–benefit' calculations could be conducted within an EMR and displayed for interventions suggested by each clinical practice guideline for an individual patient. This would allow the practitioner and the patient to make care plans based on an understanding of the implications of each intervention, given the multiple morbidities of the patient. Finally, and most importantly, the design of the EMR needs to facilitate the practitioner's treatment of the patient as a 'whole person', reflecting the goals of the patient with multimorbidity.

Conclusion

This chapter outlines five key tasks, which are necessary to achieve comprehensive use of the EMR in the care of patients with multimorbidity and identifies several areas where EMRs need to evolve to better support the care of these patients. Focusing on the future, there are three key areas of innovation and change that will be associated with the use of EMRs for patients with multimorbidity. First, through individualized access to the EMR, patients will become more engaged in accessing, changing and validating health information held in their healthcare practitioner's records or their own personal health records. Second, the evolving expectations of EMR users will result in an increased demand for EMR design that supports more efficient use and data entry. Finally, as use of EMR data continues to increase, the ability to interpret, validate and analyze data in the care of patients with multimorbidity will improve (Boxes 7.1 and 7.2).

Box 7.1 **The management of the multimorbid patient in the year 2020?**

You have known your patient John Brown for many years. He has diabetes, hypertension, asthma, atrial fibrillation and hypothyroidism and is on several medications including a blood thinner. He routinely sends you his home blood pressure and blood sugar readings taken by using his electronic measuring device securely through the Internet to your EMR. Today, you get a message from John through your EMR that he has been having some mild increase in shortness of breath over the past few days. Also, your EMR alerts you that John has a significant increase in his heart rate over the last few readings. You send a message to your nurse practitioner requesting them to review John's chart and do a home assessment. In addition, you submit an electronic request to the lab technicians to visit John's home and perform an ECG along with some blood tests. The nurse practitioner examines John at his home and uses a mobile computer to send you messages. It appears that John indeed has an increased heart rate with no other physical findings. The lab had just transmitted John's ECG into your EMR as well. The ECG reports an irregular heartbeat compatible with rapid atrial fibrillation. John does not want to go to hospital for further assessment. While awaiting the blood results, you work on getting John feeling better by getting his heart rate under control. You start to prescribe a beta blocker but your EMR warns you of a drug–disease interaction, specifically, a potential worsening of asthma with the use of beta blockers. Instead, you use a calcium channel blocker. The prescription is electronically sent to the pharmacist and the medication is quickly delivered to John's home. You monitor John more closely through his home devices and find that John's heart rate has improved the next day. John sends you a message that he is feeling better. In addition, you get an alert from your chart that John's blood work showed a significant hyperthyroid state. You talk to John by phone and find out that he has been incorrectly taking his thyroid medication with his recent medication renewal. You help him correct the problem and he thanks you for not having to go to hospital.

Box 7.2

What are the five key tasks to pay attention to in order to best use current EMRs?
How might EMRs better support the care of patients with multimorbidity in the future?

Further reading

Dawes, M. (2010) Co-morbidity: we need a guideline for each patient not a guideline for each disease. *Family Practice*, **27**, 1–2.

Guthrie, B., Payne, K., Alderson, P., McMurdo, M.E.T. & Mercer, S.W. (2012) Adapting clinical guidelines to take account of multimorbidity. *British Medical Journal*, **345**, e6341.

Ryan, B.L., Shadd, J.D., Terry, A., Cejic, S., Chevendra, V. & Thind, A. (2011) You and your EMR: the research perspective. Part 2. How structure matters. *Canadian Family Physician*, **57**, 1473–1474.

Schoen, C., Osborn, R., Squires, D. *et al.* (2012) A survey of primary care doctors in ten countries shows progress in use of health information technology, less in other areas. *Health Affairs (Millwood)*, **31** (12), 2805–2816.

Terry, A.L., Cejic, S., Ryan, B.L. *et al.* (2012) You and your EMR: the research perspective. Part four. Optimizing EMRs in primary health care practice and research. *Canadian Family Physician*, **58** (6), 705–706.

CHAPTER 8

Treatment Burden and Multimorbidity

Katie I. Gallacher[1], Victor M. Montori[2], Carl R. May[3], and Frances S. Mair[1]

[1]General Practice and Primary Care, Institute of Health and Wellbeing, University of Glasgow, UK
[2]Knowledge and Evaluation Research Unit, Department of Health Sciences Research and Medicine, Mayo Clinic, USA
[3]Faculty of Health Sciences, University of Southampton, UK

OVERVIEW

- Patients with long-term conditions experience treatment burden
- The key components of treatment burden are learning about treatments and their consequences, engaging with others, adhering to treatments and lifestyle changes and monitoring treatments
- Multimorbidity can affect patients by (1) increasing treatment burden and (2) decreasing the capacity of the patient to cope
- Excessive treatment burden can reduce adherence to management plans and lead to negative outcomes for patients and their caregivers
- Better ways of measuring treatment burden are required
- Changes are needed at practice and policy level to minimize treatment burden and improve patient outcomes among multimorbid patients.

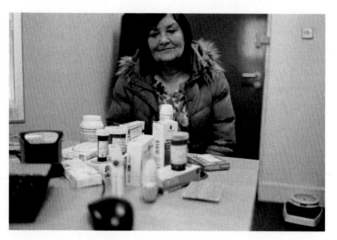

Figure 8.1 Polypharmacy is only one aspect of treatment burden but a substantial one for many patients with multimorbidity.

Definition of treatment burden

Treatment burden refers to the tasks that patients with a long-term condition must perform to respond to the requirements of their healthcare providers and the impact that these practices have on their functioning and well-being. This includes all activities that healthcare providers require those with long-term conditions to perform to manage their illness, including learning about treatments and their side effects, taking medications, enacting lifestyle changes, attending appointments, undergoing investigations and monitoring symptoms (see Figure 8.1). Treatment burden encompasses a different set of burdens to those imposed by the illness itself such as symptoms, disabilities and psychological difficulties. However, illness and treatment burden certainly influence one another and also overlap. For example, a stroke patient who is suffering from depression (illness burden) may fail to carry out the demanding daily physiotherapy exercises assigned to him (treatment burden) and therefore fail to improve physically (illness burden).

Patient capacity

Patients suffering from different types and levels of morbidity will experience different kinds of treatment burden, often as a result of management decisions taken by health professionals. The capacity that a patient has to cope with these demands will influence the patient's experience. Internal factors may include personal capabilities, level of education, personality, cognition and psychological condition; external factors may include amount of social support, employment, financial circumstances and available community facilities. As healthcare providers impose heavier treatment burden, then the capacity of patients and caregivers to accommodate these demands is stretched until a 'coping threshold' is reached, beyond which the balance tips and patients fail to follow treatments. Alternatively, patients may perceive the coping threshold approaching and unilaterally prioritize their workload in order to 'fit' their capacity and maintain a balance. Or patients with stable treatment plans may see their capacity reduced by competing demands (personal or work-related, emotional or financial, mental or physical illness) and be no longer able to sustain the current treatments (see Figure 8.2).

ABC of Multimorbidity, First Edition.
Edited by Stewart W. Mercer, Chris Salisbury and Martin Fortin.
© 2014 John Wiley & Sons, Ltd. Published 2014 by John Wiley & Sons, Ltd.

Treatment burden and multimorbidity

As we have seen in Chapter 2, multimorbidity is becoming increasingly common. Long-term conditions require lifelong management with input from health services and long-term investment from patients. Owing to advances in science and technology, patients are living longer, following more complicated management plans, utilizing more health services (Chapter 4) and therefore experiencing an increasing level of treatment burden.

Multimorbidity can affect patients by (1) increasing treatment burden and (2) decreasing the capacity of the patient to cope with these demands. Treatment burden is likely to increase with each extra morbidity not only because of an increase in the volume of tasks but also because these may actually negatively interact with each other [e.g. drug interactions (Figure 8.1) or clashing appointment times]. Recently, health services have increasingly moved away from the provision of generalized care to a more speciality-based service increasing the number of healthcare professionals involved with each patient and resulting in a more disease-centred approach. This has resulted in an increase in treatment burden for patients. As mentioned earlier, multimorbidity may decrease patient capacity as patients are more likely to suffer from a poorer quality of life and functional status (Chapter 3), as well as being more at risk of depression and psychological disorders (Chapter 9). All of these factors may decrease the patient's ability to cope with the demands of illness management.

Patient adherence and other outcomes

As discussed earlier, increasing levels of treatment burden may overwhelm the patient, pushing them past their 'coping threshold' and leading to a reduced adherence to therapies (see Figure 8.2). Non-adherence may result from patients feeling that they have too much to cope with and cutting back on aspects of care to make life more manageable. It may also result from a misunderstanding or

error by the patient as formal or informal care processes become increasingly complicated. Non-adherence in the management of long-term conditions is a global health problem identified by the World Heath Association. Non-adherence is associated with negative outcomes such as increased morbidity and mortality, difficulties in professional–patient relationships and wasted expenditure by health services. Whilst improving patient knowledge, through education and access to sources of information, positively affects adherence, there is good evidence that workload factors, including the scheduling of treatments and the logistics of access to care, can play a major role. It is therefore of vital importance that the issue of treatment burden is addressed in order to improve patient outcomes (see Figure 8.3).

Typology of treatment burden

The key components of treatment burden are learning about treatments and their consequences, engaging with others, adhering to treatments and lifestyle changes and monitoring treatments (see Figure 8.4, Box 8.1).

Box 8.1

What are the key components of treatment burden?
What are the effects of excessive treatment burden in patients with multimorbidity?
How might treatment burden be decreased in patients with multimorbidity?

Learning about treatments and their consequences

In order to follow management plans set out by health professionals, patients need to reach an adequate level of understanding of their illness and treatments. This includes understanding the importance

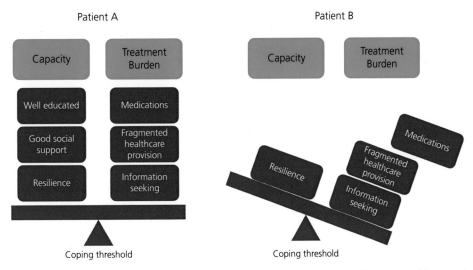

Figure 8.2 A demonstration of the balance between patient capacity and treatment burden. The two scales each represent a different patient. Patient A: treatment burden and patient capacity are balanced, the patient maintains their management plan. Patient B: treatment burden outweighs patient capacity, the coping threshold is exceeded and the balance tips leading to a collapse in the management and failure to follow treatments.

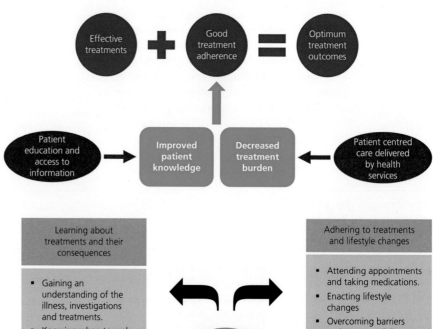

Figure 8.3 The association between knowledge, treatment burden and adherence.

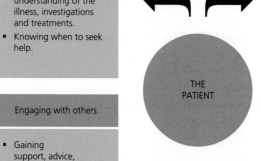

Figure 8.4 Typology of treatment burden. Gallacher *et al.* 2011.

of therapies, how to follow regimes and make lifestyle changes, what side effects may occur and when to seek help. Patients may speak to health professionals to gain information or spend time researching books, leaflets or the Internet. They spend time organizing their care, setting schedules and planning activities in advance. Patients and clinicians may also engage in shared decision-making, considering the pros and cons of therapies in light of the goals the patient may have. Patients face difficulties when information is not made available to them forcing them to work harder to gain an understanding of their treatments.

Engaging with others

Patients develop relationships with health professionals, rely on them for advice and reassurance and contact them for help when required. They also ask friends and family to provide both practical and emotional support, such as transportation to hospital, prescription collection or moral support during appointments. Patients also endure negative effects on their relationships with friends and family and protect family members from the stress of caring for them. They engage with fellow patients and attend support groups,

spending time helping others as well as gaining information and support themselves.

Adhering to treatments and lifestyle changes

Patients spend a significant amount of time and effort following medication regimes, using devices such as dosette boxes and log books to keep track of regimes and enduring unpleasant side effects. They have to enact lifestyle changes and attend multiple appointments with a range of health professionals requiring them to deal with problems stemming from lack of continuity and poor communication. Adaptations are made to the home and technical aids acquired for mobility. Treatments are integrated into their daily lives with new routines and limitations. Patients may be significantly affected financially depending on healthcare and social provision; for example, patients may have to pay for new housing or pay for health care in certain countries.

Monitoring treatments

Patients appraise therapies by monitoring changes in symptoms and progress in rehabilitation and may alter medication regimes for a variety of reasons. They make decisions about continuing regimes both on their own and in discussion with healthcare professionals. They may be up to date with new treatments available by asking their doctor and by carrying out their own research.

What can be done to identify treatment burden and lessen this for patients?

In order to lessen treatment burden for patients and improve outcomes, significant changes are needed from the policy level down to the clinical consultation. The clinical encounter plays a vital role; health professionals must consider the patient's capacity and the possible impact of treatment burden when recommending therapies.

Importantly, enhancing patient access to information and improving professional–patient encounters can make it easier for patients to reach an understanding of their therapies, vital to enable patients and caregivers to be able to organize regimes, follow management plans and appraise therapies. This may necessitate longer consultation times. Medication regimes should be simplified as much as possible. This will depend on how therapies are financed, and a balance must be achieved between cost-effective, affordable treatments and regimes that are easy to follow. For example, a change in supplier of tablets to reflect the cheapest available may confuse patients who rely on a comprehension of shape and colour when following their daily medication regime. A more complicated regime may be cheaper but money would be wasted if the patient fails to adhere to the treatments. Polypills would cut the number of tablets required, but their safety and efficacy needs to be proven before they are made widely available and the advantages for those with multimorbidity are unclear.

Care should be patient-centred rather than disease-centred to minimize the volume of appointments and therapists involved. For example, multimorbid patients may attend separate annual check-ups in primary care for each morbidity, but these appointments could be combined into one 'holistic' appointment, during which all conditions would be reviewed together, minimizing duplication and negative interactions between therapies. Similarly in secondary care, investigations and check-ups could be arranged on the same day for each patient to minimize travel to the hospital, in the form of a 'one-stop shop' for patients. Where patients receive care from different sectors, for example, from both primary and secondary care providers, communication must be adequate to optimize patient care. For example, communication between primary and secondary care after discharge from hospital is often inadequate, with a resultant chaotic and stressful period for patients. Similarly, continuity of care is extremely important to patients and can minimize duplication and medical error. Building a trusting relationship with health professionals is important for patients with multimorbidity, and maximizing continuity of care would make this easier (see Chapter 5).

Gaps in knowledge

There is a lack of research in examining the patient's experience of treatment burden in long-term conditions, particularly in patients with multimorbidity. Recent research has concentrated on chronic heart failure, stroke, diabetes and chronic kidney disease, but other conditions must be examined and multimorbidity explored. To move forward, we need to use both qualitative and quantitative research to identify different aspects of treatment burden as well as intervention points and enable the development of a measurement method that could be used in the clinical consultation. The full extent of treatment burden experienced by patients with multimorbidity is not yet known. Such knowledge will inform required changes at both practice and policy level in order to minimize treatment burden and improve patient outcomes.

Acknowledgements

We would like to acknowledge The International Minimally Disruptive Medicine Workgroup, which includes Victor M. Montori, Carl R. May, Frances S. Mair, Katie I. Gallacher, David T. Eton, Deborah Morrison, Bhautesh Jani, Sara Macdonald, Susan Browne, David Blane, Nilay Shah, Nathan Shipee, Patricia Erwin and Kathleen Yost.

Further reading

Bayliss, E.A., Steiner, J.F., Crane, L.A. & Main, D.S. (2003) Descriptions of barriers to self-care by persons with comorbid chronic diseases. *Annals of Family Medicine*, **1** (1), 15–21.

Bohlen, K., Scoville, E., Shippee, N.D., May, C.R. & Montori, V.M. (2012) Overwhelmed patients: a videographic analysis of how patients and clinicians articulate and address treatment burden during clinical encounters. *Diabetes Care*, **35** (1), 47–49.

Gallacher, K., May, C., Montori, V.M. & Mair, F.S. (2011) Understanding treatment burden in chronic heart failure patients. A qualitative study. *Annals of Family Medicine*, **9**, 235–243.

Gallacher, K., Morrison, D., Jani, B. *et al.* (2013) Uncovering Treatment Burden as a Key Concept for Stroke Care: A Systematic Review of Qualitative Research. PLoS Med 10: 10.1371/journal.pmed.1001473.

Haynes, R.B., McDonald, H.P. & Garg, A.X. (2002) Helping patients follow prescribed treatment: clinical applications. *Journal of the American Medical Association*, **288** (22), 2880–2883.

May, C., Montori, V.M. & Mair, F.S. (2009) We need minimally disruptive medicine. *British Medical Journal*, **339**, b2803.

Shippee, N.D., Shah, N.D., May, C.R., Mair, F.S. & Montori, V.M. (2012) Cumulative complexity: a functional, patient centred model of patient complexity can improve research and practice. *Journal of Clinical Epidemiology*, **65** (10), 1041–1051.

Tinetti, M.E., Fried, T.R. & Boyd, C.M. (2012) Designing health care for the mostcommon chronic condition – multimorbidity. *Journal of the American Medical Association*, **307** (23), 2493–2494.

Eduardo Sabaté *World Health Organization adherence to long-term therapies – evidence for action* (2003) http://apps.who.int/medicinedocs/en/d/Js4883e/5.html ISBN 92 4 154599 2

CHAPTER 9

Multimorbidity and Mental Health

Peter Bower[1], Peter Coventry[2], Linda Gask[1], and Jane Gunn[3]

[1]Centre for Primary Care, NIHR School for Primary Care Research, Manchester Academic Health Science Centre, University of Manchester, UK
[2]NIHR CLAHRC for Greater Manchester, Manchester Academic Health Science Centre, University of Manchester, Manchester, UK
[3]Department of General Practice and Primary Health Care, Academic Centre Melbourne Medical School, The University of Melbourne

---

OVERVIEW

- Patients with long-term conditions have a high prevalence of problems such as depression and anxiety
- The presence of depression and anxiety can have significant implications for self-management of long-term conditions and quality of life
- There are important barriers to the recognition and management of depression and anxiety in patients with long-term conditions
- The management of depression and anxiety in patients with long-term conditions may be improved through the adoption of common principles of 'chronic disease management' and 'collaborative care'.

Background

This chapter considers what is known about multimorbidity when long term conditions and mental health problems coexist and explores the challenges faced by clinicians and services to respond to the needs of patients.

Common mental health problems and long-term conditions

As Moussavi *et al.* (2007) have found, patients with long-term conditions have a high prevalence of major depressive illness. The co-occurrence of long-term conditions and mental health problems is shown in Figure 9.1. Many patients, like John in the case study in Box 9.1, may attribute the cause of their depression to reaction to a long-term condition and the limitations that it brings. However, depression and long-term conditions share a complex relationship. Long-term conditions can lead to depression, but depression is also an important risk factor for later long-term conditions. Less attention has been given to anxiety even though symptoms of anxiety and depression are highly correlated, and 'mixed anxiety and depression' is very common in primary care.

ABC of Multimorbidity, First Edition.
Edited by Stewart W. Mercer, Chris Salisbury and Martin Fortin.
© 2014 John Wiley & Sons, Ltd. Published 2014 by John Wiley & Sons, Ltd.

Box 9.1 Case example – depression and long-term conditions

John is a 48-year-old labourer with coronary heart disease. John has put on weight and is not adherent with his medication, and his nurse is concerned that he is putting himself at risk. His general practitioner (GP) conducts a mental health assessment, including the Patient Health Questionnaire 9 (PHQ 9), which is a short self-report measure of depressive symptoms.

His PHQ 9 score is 19, indicating moderately severe depression. Although John accepts that the PHQ score is a fair reflection of the way he feels, he is resistant when the term 'depression' is mentioned. He does not feel that he has a 'mental illness' and states categorically that the way he feels reflects the impact of coronary heart disease on his work and personal life, and his everyday pleasures such as drinking and smoking. He feels that it is these issues that are making him feel down, and if there were better ways of managing his heart problems, the feelings would disappear.

The clinical implications of common mental health problems in long-term conditions

Irrespective of controversies over cause and effect, the major concern of clinicians is on the impact of mental health and long-term conditions on patient experience, mortality and morbidity, and quality of life.

The UK Department of Health defines self-management as 'the care taken by individuals towards their own health and well being' and includes a healthy lifestyle, social and emotional needs, managing the condition and prevention. Depression can reduce motivation and capacity for self-management and poor outcomes in people with comorbid depression alongside long-term conditions such as diabetes may reflect poor self-management. Patients with depression may have a feeling of hopelessness (which may influence feelings about treatment effectiveness), may be more likely to be socially isolated and lacking support and may struggle with limited concentration and energy. Sometimes, the management of one condition actively conflicts with the management of another. For example, treating a depressed patient might lead to a better mood but that might lead to a return of their appetite with potential negative effects on diet and diabetes care.

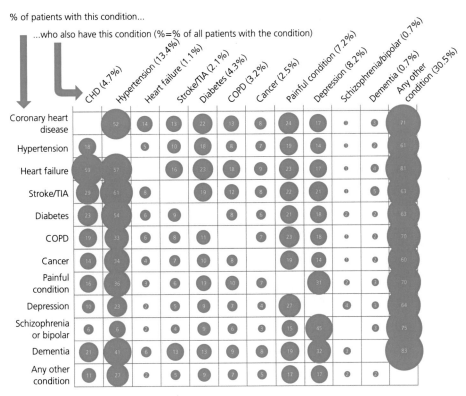

Figure 9.1 Co-occurrence of physical and mental conditions in primary care patients. Source: Barnett *et al*. 2012. Reproduced with permission of Elsevier.

Equally important is the potential for the management of the long-term condition to have an impact on mood. Patients with long-term conditions are expected to monitor symptoms and make changes to their lifestyle, and many patients might find such activities to have a significant impact on their quality of life. Patients with multimorbidity have to deal with many self-management activities with only limited resources of energy, time, attention and motivation. This has led to calls for clinicians to think about not only the burden of disease in such patients but also the burden of treatment (see Chapter 8).

The organization of the healthcare system may contribute to the problem. Some aspects of the management of depression are better in patients with long-term conditions because the routine follow-up of patients with long-term conditions increases the opportunity to effectively manage depression, and single interventions can confer benefits for multiple disorders (e.g., exercise prescribed for the control of diabetes may impact favourably on mood).

However, the presence of mental and physical health multimorbidity can be problematic for a variety of reasons. The time-limited nature of primary care consultations means that decision-making is often centred around immediate patient concerns. Opportunities to offer patients an integrated approach to care, responding to physical and mental health problems are limited. Competing demands on health professional time often leads to priority being given to physical health problems. Those priorities are often reflected in patient behaviour as well.

It is possible that patients with comorbid depression and long-term conditions have difficulty in communicating effectively with practitioners. People with depression may not be active

in seeking care at certain points in their lives, especially when symptoms are severe. In the presence of long-term conditions, both health professionals and patients *normalize* depression as a natural consequence of symptoms and loss of function. Even where health professionals are skilled at detecting depression, our case study (Box 9.1) highlights the difficulties in negotiating labels and treatment strategies with patients who may attribute symptoms of depression to other causes. Practitioners may avoid discussing self-management because they feel it might upset or annoy the patient.

A UK primary care study (Coventry *et al*. 2011; see Box 9.2) that examined barriers to depression care in multimorbidity found that recognition of depression is difficult. Depression can be misconstrued as part of ageing. If depressive symptoms appear periodically, there may be greater focus on physical problems.

In discussing mental health, patients with multimorbidity are acutely aware of the stigma associated with depressive illness, delaying help-seeking. In response to this, some have highlighted the benefits of using non-psychiatric language with patients with multimorbidity and how drawing on metaphors and figurative language can help patients to discuss their emotional health in less stigmatizing ways.

Management of long-term conditions – the chronic care model and collaborative care

The burden of long-term conditions and multimorbidity has led to important innovations in the delivery of care, such as the chronic care model (described in earlier chapters). In mental health, an equally important influence on the delivery of care has been the adoption of stepped care models. This model is based on two core principles. Patients with less severe depression are initially given low-intensity interventions, such as written self-help and computerized forms of treatments. They are only 'stepped-up' to high-intensity (and more costly) treatments if they fail to benefit. All patients are followed up regularly in stepped care systems to ensure that they achieve appropriate outcomes and are 'stepped-up' if necessary.

Integrating management of depression into care for long-term conditions

One of the problems with the standard approaches to managing depression is that they are oriented to manage depression as an acute problem. This means that patients seek help when they deem it necessary, and professionals respond to those patients seeking help, rather than considering the needs of the wider population. This makes little sense when it is known that depressed patients may not be motivated to seek care. This had led to the interest in the adoption of the chronic care model to improve quality and outcomes in depression.

Long-term conditions and depression – the collaborative care model

The management of depression has been revolutionized by the emergence of 'collaborative care'. This innovation has primarily

been led by Katon and Unützer (2010) in the USA. Collaborative care shares the broad philosophy of the chronic care model and suggests that the changes in the organization and delivery of services that are required for disorders such as diabetes and arthritis are of equal relevance to depression. The nature of collaborative care models varies, but Box 9.3 provides a case history based on a UK model of collaborative care for depression and vascular disease, which is currently being evaluated.

Severe mental illness and long-term conditions

Severe mental illnesses (such as psychoses) are less prevalent than depression or anxiety, but the physical health needs of these patients cannot be ignored. As explored by Chang *et al.* (2011), people with severe mental illness are at considerably greater risk of having comorbid physical health problems and die 10–15 years earlier than when compared with the general population. The reasons for this are complex. Some of these effects are related to lifestyle as such patients may be less likely to exercise, and more likely to have a poor diet, and to smoke and drink excessively. They may also have poor access to health care partly as a result of 'diagnostic overshadowing' (in which the diagnosis of severe mental health problems obscures other problems) and partly because of reduced likelihood of routine screening. Finally, there is the impact of medication, which may lead to a significant weight gain and a higher risk of diabetes and metabolic syndrome.

Management of long-term conditions in coexisting severe mental illness

Guidance for patients with schizophrenia emphasizes the need to focus on cardiovascular risk, and for close liaison between primary and specialist care (see Box 9.4). Primary healthcare professionals should monitor the physical health of people with schizophrenia at least once a year, and results should be sent to the care co-ordinator or psychiatrist and placed in notes in specialist settings.

Box 9.4 **Case example – severe mental illness and long-term conditions**

Julie is a 28-year-old woman who was diagnosed with schizophrenia about five years ago. At that time, she became acutely psychotic and was detained in a hospital. She began her treatment with antipsychotic medication and is currently taking olanzapine 10 mg. Her mental state has improved considerably during this time but she has put on a great deal of weight and her mother is concerned that she has stopped going out because she feels very conscious of her appearance. She is also smoking very heavily, 20–30 cigarettes per day.

She has a key worker in the mental health team whom she sees once a month. She does not like going to see her GP because she hates sitting in the waiting room where she thinks people stare at her. However, she has recently been sent a letter asking her to attend her annual health check at the practice. She is not sure if she is going to attend.

However, despite the increasing focus on addressing physical health, there remain a proportion of people with severe mental illness who do not attend primary care and are difficult to engage and motivate. There is also sometimes a confusion about whether the mental health team or the GP should follow-up abnormal results, and whether negotiation is required between mental health and primary care services to ensure clarity of arrangements. It would seem appropriate that during the acute and continuation phase of mental health care, follow-up of abnormal results should be the responsibility of the main mental health professional providing care, unless there has been an agreed delegation; but treatment should be provided by an appropriate practitioner who is skilled and confident to do so.

Therapeutic nihilism in the management of long-term conditions in serious mental illness is misplaced. As with depression, more comprehensive strategies may employ a 'collaborative care' approach working closely with physical healthcare providers, as discussed by Druss *et al.* (2010).

In general medical settings, it is important to remember that people with dementia and other types of cognitive impairment may have difficulty conveying their distress and communicating experience such as pain. Unhelpful attitudes towards mental illness and

learning difficulty may also mean that attempts have not been made to try and help people who might require physical health care. Attitudes towards substance misuse may result in poor care for the physical complications which are often present.

In the case example (Box 9.4), it is clear that Julie will need support from her key worker to attend her health check, and good communication between GP and mental health services is needed to ensure this. Julie may benefit from referral for help with both her smoking and weight; however, both her key worker and GP will need to help to motivate her to engage with this support. It is essential that they help her to see how doing this will both help her to feel better about herself and to lead a healthier and longer life (Box 9.5).

Box 9.5

In what ways might mental and health problems interact in patients with multimorbidity?
What models of care may help patients with mental–physical multimorbidity and how do they work?

Further reading

Barnett, K., Mercer, S., Norbury, M. *et al.* (2012) Epidemiology of multimorbidity and implications for health care, research, and medical education: a cross-sectional study. *Lancet*, **380** (9836), 37–43.

Chang, C., Hayes, R., Perera, G. *et al.* (2011) Life expectancy at birth for people with serious mental illness and other major disorders from a secondary mental health care case register in London. *Plos ONE*, **6**, e19590.

Coventry, P., Hays, R., Dickens, C. *et al.* (2011) Talking about depression: a qualitative study of barriers to managing depression in people with long term conditions in primary care. *BMC Family Practice*, **12**, 10.

Druss, B., von Esenwein, S., Compton, M., Rask, K., Zhao, L. & Parker, R. (2010) A randomized trial of medical care management for community mental health settings: the Primary Care Access, Referral, and Evaluation (PCARE) study. *The American Journal of Psychiatry*, **167**, 151–159.

Katon, W. & Unützer, J. (2010) Collaborative care models for depression: time to move from evidence to practice. *Archives of Internal Medicine*, **166**, 2304–2306.

Moussavi, S., Chatterji, S., Verdes, E., Tandon, A., Patel, V. & Ustun, B. (2007) Depression, chronic diseases, and decrements in health: results from the World Health Surveys. *Lancet*, **370**, 851–858.

National Institute for Health and Clinical Excellence (2009) Depression in adults with a chronic physical health problem: treatment and management (National Clinical Practice Guideline Number 91). http://www.nice.org.uk/nicemedia/pdf/CG91FullGuideline.pdf

National Institute for Health and Clinical Excellence (2011) NICE Guideline 82 Schizophrenia. http://www.nice.org.uk/nicemedia/live/11786/43607/43607.pdf

Naylor, C., Parsonage, M., McDaid, D., Knapp, M., Fossey, M. & Galea, A. (2012) Long-Term Conditions and Mental Health. The Cost of Co-Morbidities. King's Fund and Centre for Mental Health, London.

Royal College of Psychiatrists *Improving physical and mental health*. http://www.rcpsych.ac.uk/mentalhealthinfo/improvingphysicalandmh.aspx. accessed 16 March 2014

CHAPTER 10

The Impact of Multimorbidity on Quality and Safety of Health Care

Jose M. Valderas[1,2,3,4], *Ignacio Ricci-Cabello*[3], *and Concepción Violán*[3,4]

[1]Health Services and Policy Research Group, Department of Primary Care Health Sciences, University of Oxford, UK
[2]LSE Health, London School of Economics and Political Science, UK
[3]Institut Universitari d'Investigació en Atenció Primària Jordi Gol (IDIAP Jordi Gol), Spain
[4]Universitat Autònoma de Barcelona, Spain

OVERVIEW

- Multimorbidity has the potential for resulting in poor quality of care and increased threats to patient safety. Multimorbidity has been associated with better quality of care as measured by the combination of condition-specific indicators but worse care when assessed from a patient-centred perspective
- No study has focused on the evaluation of patient safety in multimorbidity
- There is a need for conceptual clarity in future assessments and for the development of valid and reliable indicators of quality and safety in multimorbidity, including the recognition that quality of care for these patients requires more than delivering care that is consistent with the current disease-specific guidelines
- Clinicians should apply caution when delivering care for these patients in the absence of evidence for the benefits and harm of available management options
- Health systems should focus on enhancing primary care-centred coordination and continuity of care and designing incentives systems that reward appropriate care for these patients.

Introduction

The fact that a significant proportion of patients suffer from multimorbidity induces a tension between a healthcare model centred around the patient and health services that are organized around the diagnosis and management of individual health conditions. This tension has the potential for resulting in poor quality of care and threats to patient safety.

In this chapter, we review the key concepts for understanding the potentially detrimental effects of multimorbidity on quality and safety along with the opportunities for beneficial effects, the evidence for the impact of multimorbidity on quality and safety of care, how discrepancies between different studies can be reconciled and discuss the implications for providing care for multimorbid patients.

ABC of Multimorbidity, First Edition.
Edited by Stewart W. Mercer, Chris Salisbury and Martin Fortin.
© 2014 John Wiley & Sons, Ltd. Published 2014 by John Wiley & Sons, Ltd.

Key theoretical issues on the impact of multimorbidity on quality and safety of health care

Quality of care has been traditionally considered to be a characteristic of the process of healthcare delivery, as assessed in relation to standards. Ideally, there should be empirical evidence that care that adheres to such standards contributes to the delivery of efficient and effective health care. We will use the same approach for defining patient safety as a characteristic of the process of care delivery oriented towards the minimization of harm resulting from the interaction with the health system.

Multimorbidity might have potentially detrimental effects on quality and safety. People suffering from multiple health conditions are more likely to require an increased number of healthcare processes (Boyd *et al.*, 2005), which will also trigger the involvement of an increased number of health professionals. This increased complexity in the delivery of care may threaten coordination, continuity and safety, thereby decreasing the likelihood of receiving care that meets high standards of quality and safety. Alternatively, it may be argued that the increased interaction with the health services might well result in increased opportunities for receiving effective care and also that the intrinsic high-risk profile of these patients might result in an increased patient safety awareness by the health professional involved.

There is no doubt that the quality and safety of patients with multimorbidity must take into account the evidence for the management of each individual condition. High quality and safe care for a patient with hypertension, osteoarthritis and chronic obstructive pulmonary disease must be informed by best practice guidelines for each of high blood pressure, osteoarthritis and chronic obstructive pulmonary disease. But it is also important to stress here that it must *also* incorporate considerations about multimorbidity itself and its implications for management. We can hardly speak of safe high-quality care for this patient if the potentially antagonistic goals are not adequately addressed, interactions between the corresponding medications are not carefully examined (see Figure 10.1) and adequate coordination does not ensure smooth follow-up and monitoring of each of the conditions *and* the health status of the patient, including liaising with the corresponding specialists, while at the same time avoiding overexposing the patient to unnecessary health care and their potential or actual complications. And yet, as

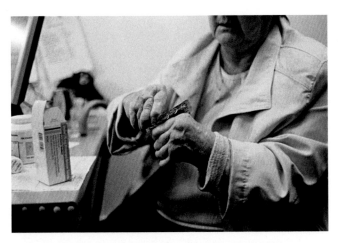

Figure 10.1 Little is known about safety of care in patients with multimorbidity, but iatrogenesis related to polypharmacy is an obvious area for concern.

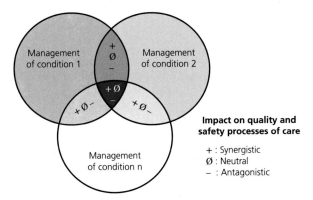

Impact on quality and safety processes of care

+ : Synergistic
Ø : Neutral
– : Antagonistic

Figure 10.2 Impact of multimorbidity on quality and safety.

we will see, all these issues have been grossly overlooked, restricting evaluations in most cases to the specifics of care for each separate condition.

The management of concurrent health conditions may benefit from synergies when the conditions share a patho-physiological pathway. However, given any pair of conditions, their simultaneous management may be enhanced, impaired or simply not be affected, which can be termed as synergistic, antagonistic and neutral combinations (Valderas *et al.* 2009). This would separately apply to each specific management process (diagnosis, treatment, monitoring, etc.), and this may result in overall interactions between conditions that are not necessarily purely synergistic, antagonistic or neutral but rather mixed (see Figure 10.2). This is the reason why this approach to classifying interaction has been almost exclusively applied to a specific cluster of cardiovascular conditions, including coronary heart disease, diabetes, hypertension, hypercholesterolemia and peripheral artery disease, where all the interactions are of the same nature.

Evidence for the impact of multimorbidity on the quality and safety of health care

Evidence on this issue is scarce. Just two studies have specifically studied the impact of multimorbidity on the quality of care, and no

studies have focussed on the issue of patient safety in this highly vulnerable population, or at least it has not been addressed as a clearly distinct issue.

The most comprehensive study so far was conducted in the USA by Higashi *et al.* (2007) and included three large independent datasets. Researchers found that the overall quality of care, as measured using a database of several hundreds, mostly disease-specific indicators, increased with the number of comorbid conditions, and this relationship was maintained after controlling for the numbers of visits. In another study, multimorbidity was inversely associated with communication ratings. Ten groups of synergistic combinations of conditions were hypothesized, and the number of different groups in each patient showed a similar pattern of association with poor communication (Fung *et al.* 2008).

Although the picture that emerges is somewhat fuzzy because of the lack of a consistent approach and the somewhat contradictory results, it would appear that multimorbidity seems to be associated with worse quality of care when measured using a patient-centred approach. As for patient safety, the lack of evidence makes it impossible to draw any inference.

The main limitation of these studies is that they have failed to use indicators of quality of care (and patient safety) that are specific to the care of patients with multimorbidity. But the onus is not necessarily on these researchers. We simply lack well-validated and established indicators that are fit for this purpose. Out of the several hundreds of indicators used in the study by Higashi *et al.*, none was specific for multimorbidity. The Quality and Outcomes Framework in the UK does not include at present any indicator specific for patients with multimorbidity, nor do the Quality Indicators used by the Agency for Healthcare Research and Quality in the USA.

Implications for clinical practice

Clinical guidelines constitute the reference for the clinical management of patients, but, the applicability of current evidence-based guidelines to multimorbid patients is limited and can be problematic. This raises the fundamental question of whether not providing guidelines consistent care for people with multimorbidity represents poor quality care (an assumption made by all previous studies) or whether it actually reflects care that is sensitive to the particular needs of these patients (Box 10.1).

Box 10.1

Patients with multimorbidity have frequent contacts with multiple healthcare providers. Does this lead to better or worse care?
When is it appropriate for healthcare professionals to ignore the chronic disease treatment guidelines?
How can we define and measure improved outcomes in multimorbidity?

However, a more patient-centred approach, is one where the aim is to improve the quality of care with the patient as the framework of reference, and here it is clear that the whole approach is more than the sum of the parts. Quality of care for a patient with multiple conditions is more than just the sum of the components of quality of care for the individual conditions. What is relevant is how all the threads (care for each condition from which an individual suffers) are spun into a yarn (care for the individual). A recent systematic review has shed some light on what might constitute effective care for patients with multimorbidity (Smith *et al.* 2012). It has also made evident the paucity of interventions that have demonstrated some benefit for patients with multimorbidity. Organizational interventions that target specific risk factors or areas where patients may have difficulties (such as with functional ability or medicine management), seem more likely to be effective. Other organizational interventions with a broader focus (notably case management or changes in care delivery) or patient-oriented interventions that are not linked to healthcare delivery appear to be less effective. Although replication of these findings is very much needed before multimorbidity can be approached effectively, these findings provide some evidence for what can be considered to constitute high quality of care for patients with multimorbidity. In relation to patient safety, we simply need studies that illuminate the nature of the association in order to design and test effective interventions.

Clinicians should approach the management of patients with multimorbidity very much as they would approach the management of any given group of patients (defined in terms of condition, age, gender and other relevant variables) weighing up the evidence supporting any recommendations for that particular group. If there ever was a dichotomy between art and science in medicine, this is clearly an area where clinical practice is closer to the former than to the latter. The principles of minimally disruptive medicine (May *et al.*, 2009) might provide helpful guidance for decision-making decisions in everyday practice for patients with multimorbidity (see Chapter 8).

Efforts should be made to ensure that continuity and coordination of care for these patients is ensured. Interestingly, the evidence suggests that complex models of care (such as case management) do not necessarily pay off, making use of already available alternatives, such as the enhancement of primary care services, which is a valid and potentially more efficient response.

Conclusions

Although patients with multimorbidity would be in theory at a higher risk of patient safety events and receiving poor quality of care, the evidence is inconsistent and suggests that there may also be potential benefits of current arrangements for the delivery of care. Indicators of the quality and safety of health care that are based on available evidence are very much needed before progress can be made in this field. Clinicians should apply caution when delivering care for these patients in the absence of evidence for the benefits and harm of available management options. Health systems should focus on enhancing primary care-centred coordination and continuity of care and designing incentives systems that reward appropriate care for these patients.

Acknowledgements

The authors are members of *Threads and Yarns*, a research network that draws together and provides peer support to primary care researchers across several European countries with a common interest in research for informing the provision of best health care for people with a complex clinical status.

Further reading

Boyd, C.M., Darer, J., Boult, C., Fried, L.P., Boult, L. & Wu, A.W. (2005) Clinical practice guidelines and quality of care for older patients with multiple comorbid diseases: implications for pay for performance. *Journal of the American Medical Association*, **294** (6), 716–724. doi:10.1001/jama.294.6.716

Fung, C.H., Setodji, C.M., Kung, F.-Y. *et al.* (2008) The relationship between multimorbidity and patients' ratings of communication. *Journal of General Internal Medicine*, **23** (6), 788–793. doi:10.1007/s11606-008-0602-4

Higashi, T., Wenger, N.S., Adams, J.L. *et al.* (2007) Relationship between number of medical conditions and quality of care. *New England Journal of Medicine*, **356** (24), 2496–2504. doi:10.1056/NEJMsa066253

May, C., Montori, V.M. & Mair, F.S. (11 August 2009) We need minimally disruptive medicine. *British Medical Journal*, **339**, b2803.

Smith, S.M., Soubhi, H., Fortin, M., Hudon, C. & O'Dowd, T. (3 September 2012) Managing patients with multimorbidity: systematic review of interventions in primary care and community settings. *British Medical Journal*, **345**, e5205.

Valderas, J.M., Starfield, B., Sibbald, B., Salisbury, C. & Roland, M. (2009) Defining comorbidity: implications for understanding health and health services. *Annals of Family Medicine*, **7** (4), 357–363. doi:10.1370/afm.983

CHAPTER 11

Implications of Multimorbidity for Health Policy

Chris Salisbury[1] *and Martin Roland*[2]

[1]Centre for Academic Primary Care, NIHR School for Primary Care Research, School of Social and Community Medicine, University of Bristol, UK
[2]University of Cambridge, The Primary Care Unit, Institute of Public Health, UK

OVERVIEW

- A large and increasing proportion of the population have multimorbidity, yet healthcare systems are designed as if people have only one problem at a time
- Attempts to redesign health care to reflect the needs of patients with multimorbidity would have wide implications for how we organize the system at national, regional and local levels
- Changes include valuing generalism as much as specialism, avoiding fragmentation of primary care, ensuring greater relational continuity of care, investment in shared electronic record systems and balancing vertical integration of care across primary/secondary care for individual diseases with horizontal integration of care for people with multiple diseases
- Research is needed to test new models of healthcare organization designed to address the needs of people with multimorbidity.

Background

As we have seen in the previous chapters, multimorbidity is common and its prevalence is strongly related to age. As the population ages, the number of people with multimorbidity in the population is increasing. The number of times that people consult doctors is associated with the number of health problems they have, so people with multimorbidity account for a high and increasing proportion of all consultations in primary care (Figure 11.1). In one recent study (Salisbury *et al.* 2011), 16% of people registered with GPs had more than one of the chronic conditions included in the English Quality and Outcomes Framework, but they accounted for 32% of all general practice consultations.

Many consultations in primary care therefore involve people who have multimorbidity. It is also recognized that most consultations in general practice involve the discussion of several different problems. Typical consultations in the UK general practice included discussion of an average of 2.5 different problems and several associated issues across a wide range of disease areas (Salisbury *et al.* 2013).

ABC of Multimorbidity, First Edition.
Edited by Stewart W. Mercer, Chris Salisbury and Martin Fortin.
© 2014 John Wiley & Sons, Ltd. Published 2014 by John Wiley & Sons, Ltd.

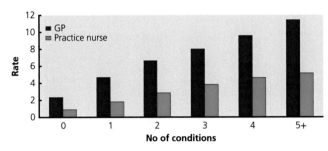

Figure 11.1 Number of consultations in general practice per year by number of chronic conditions included in the Quality and Outcomes Framework.

And yet medical care, particularly in hospital, tends to be organized as if people have only one disease at a time.

There has been a long-term trend for health care in hospitals to become increasingly specialized. There is now a similar trend in general practice towards organizing care within specific disease domains. As a means of improving the quality and consistency of care for individual conditions and to improve integration across primary and secondary care, attention has been given to creating 'disease pathways' for common chronic conditions. Processes of ideal care are clearly mapped out and protocols developed to ensure that care is systematic, efficient and coordinated. In general practice, patients are invited to specific appointments during which their chronic condition, such as diabetes or asthma, is reviewed. They often see practice nurses who have extra training in that condition and who provide care following computerized disease-specific templates based on national guidelines. The disease pathway approach seeks to improve integration of services across primary and secondary care; for example, through shared records, liaison nurses and shared protocols for care.

Therefore, there is a tension between these two opposing trends – most medical care involves managing patients with multimorbidity, and yet it is increasingly organized within single-disease pathways (Box 11.1).

Problems of the single-disease paradigm for patients

From a patient's point of view, care provided along single-disease lines is inconvenient because it often involves attending different

Box 11.1

What are the consequences of the tension between increasing specialization within primary care and the rising prevalence of multimorbidity for patients and for the healthcare system?
What would be the implications for policy of trying to design health care to suit the needs of the people who need and use it most – that is, people with multimorbidity?

clinics to discuss each of their problems. At these clinics, health professionals focus on optimizing care for one disease, which may not be the patient's top priority. Patients find it frustrating to be repeatedly asked the same questions by different health professionals, who do not seem to be very aware of their other problems and appointments, and then to be given conflicting advice (Bayliss *et al.* 2008) (Box 11.2).

Box 11.2 **What do patients say they want?**

- Better access to care by phone, email and face-to-face
- A single coordinator of care
- Continuity of care from a limited number of healthcare professionals
- Clear communication of a care plan
- Healthcare professionals to listen to and take account of their own individual needs
- Not to have protocols inflexibly applied to them

If each disease is treated in isolation, patients risk being subjected to more and more interventions each time they attend a disease-specific appointment. In order to gain optimal disease control, additional drugs may be prescribed, patients may be given other non-drug advice (such as specific exercises) and may have additional blood tests and other investigations. For people with multiple long-term conditions, this has the potential to lead to a level of intervention which is excessively complex and burdensome. Decisions often need to be made about the most important priorities, and this is difficult to do in the context of single-disease clinics. Making these judgements can be difficult as evidence about the benefits of particular treatments in patients with multimorbidity is often lacking.

However, it is important to remember how this situation has evolved. The development of guidelines, templates and clinics for conditions such as diabetes occurred because of evidence that quality of care for patients with long-term conditions was variable and sometimes poor. The introduction of these systems, incentivized by pay for performance schemes such as the Quality and Outcomes Framework in the UK, has probably helped to drive up quality and reduce inequalities in care. And although we know that patients express a desire for more holistic care from a known and trusted doctor, they express an even stronger wish to have a thorough examination and to see a professional with expertise in their health condition. So is there a way of maintaining the benefits

of systematic organized care, without losing the personal care and sense of being treated as a 'whole patient' that patients value?

Implications of multimorbidity for the healthcare system

A systems approach to the management of long-term conditions

Considerable attention has been paid to the importance of a whole-system approach to improving the management of chronic disease. The chronic care model (Epping-Jordan *et al.* 2004) has delineated a range of important factors which need to be addressed to promote effective management of chronic disease. This highlights that in order to improve care, we must not only seek to enable patients to manage their own health better through individual consultations but also ensure that structural changes are effected; for example, in how care is provided and through improved decision support and information systems.

Integrating primary and secondary care

It is widely recognized that healthcare systems that provide effective and efficient care for people with long-term conditions need to have a strong primary care foundation, which provides easily accessible generalist care and a gateway to specialist care. The important coordinating role of primary care, with judicious use of specialists, is particularly relevant to patients with multiple chronic conditions because of the risk of over-investigation and over-treatment.

However, the disadvantages of a rigid, structural divide between generalist primary care and specialist secondary care have been increasingly recognized. Primary care practitioners need easier access to specialist advice about individual patients. Specialists also have an important role in providing training, protocol development and system design. These developments are hindered by financial systems which lead to competition between primary and secondary care and create inappropriate incentives to treat patients in the wrong setting, especially if there are financial incentives on general practitioners to limit referrals to specialist care.

Promoting continuity of care

It is likely to be more efficient and more acceptable to patients if a limited number of doctors and nurses working in a small team see people with complex problems. This will increase the likelihood that the healthcare providers will be able to make decisions with a good understanding of the patient's situation and other problems and priorities. It also promotes the development of trust between patients and professionals, which is associated with greater patient satisfaction and increased adherence to treatment recommendations.

On the other hand, it is challenging for an individual clinician to be an expert in a wide range of conditions. This model of continuity from a small number of multi-skilled primary care professionals requires investment in decision support systems to prompt clinicians to provide care of consistently high quality, backed by audit systems to ensure that this quality is maintained. It also requires a careful judgement about which things are best managed by generalists (arguably, conditions which are common, such as asthma, hypertension and depression), which are better managed by specialists (those which are rare or require facilities not economically provided in the community) and which require coordination by a generalist but with occasional intervention from specialists for specific purposes (e.g., intensive short-term intervention by a specialist nurse for a patient with poorly controlled diabetes).

We know that many patients value continuity of care, but continuity is also important for reasons that patients may not appreciate. It is particularly important for patients with multiple problems: such patients are very difficult to manage in short general practice consultations if the doctor does not have prior knowledge of the patient. For these patients, continuity of care is likely to lead to better use of healthcare resources, because in a fragmented system each new doctor tends to repeat investigations 'just in case', and continuity is also likely to lead to more appropriate judgements about diagnosis and treatment. Most importantly, patients with multimorbidity need a single, clearly designated healthcare professional who is accountable for coordinating their overall management, and this requires continuity of care.

Avoiding fragmentation of primary care

It is important that patients with multimorbidity have a single point of access to the healthcare system for most of their problems, most of the time. In many countries, people have direct access to specialists. This can be advantageous for people with single, well-defined problems. But for people with multimorbidity, this is likely to lead to poorly coordinated care. Because each specialist provider cannot address all of their problems, patients with multimorbidity frequently have to be cross-referred to other providers.

Within primary care, recent policies in many countries have encouraged the development of new types of providers of primary care with the aim of promoting patient choice, encouraging competition between providers and improving access to health care. For example, the NHS in the UK has introduced walk-in centres, which offer nurse-led advice and treatment without an appointment. However, this type of care can be inefficient because of duplication of effort, leading to poor coordination of care, undermining the development of trusting relationships with health professionals and risking confusion for patients (Figure 11.2).

We should recognize that these multiple providers have often arisen because of deficiencies in the service provided by general practices, particularly in terms of access to care. However, it is likely to be more effective and efficient to improve access to general practice than to develop multiple alternative providers.

There may be benefits from having multiple providers of primary care in terms of improving access to care, but these benefits need to be balanced against a reduction in continuity and coordination of care. The balance between these advantages and disadvantages may be different for different groups of the population. For example, young people with few previous health problems, who rarely consult doctors and have busy working lives, may appreciate the convenience of walk-in centres. But the people with the biggest health needs are those with multimorbidity, and they are disadvantaged by a policy of investment in multiple new sources of care rather than

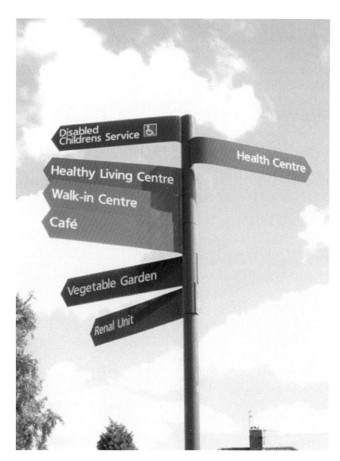

Figure 11.2 Multiple sources of care can be confusing and risks duplication.

in improved provision from a single, local, healthcare provider who is able to provide first contact generalist care for all their problems in one place and at one time.

Shared records

To some extent, the problem of patients with multimorbidity attending different specialists for each of their problems can be reduced if all the different healthcare providers have a shared system of electronic medical records. Achieving this should be a high priority for any health system that seeks to provide integrated care for people with multimorbidity, so that each care provider can take account of investigations and treatments provided elsewhere. However, the difficulties of creating a system of shared records should not be under-estimated, given the very different record-keeping needs of the different types of healthcare professionals and provider organizations within a large and complex healthcare service. Furthermore, although shared records are likely to be very important in order to promote coordination of care, it should not be assumed that a so-called 'information continuity' is a substitute for personal, relational, continuity with a known and trusted clinician.

Promoting generalist skills

If patients are able to attend one healthcare facility as the first point of contact for almost all of their health problems and if it is important to encourage continuity of care from a small number of professionals, it follows that these professionals must have an understanding of a wide range of diseases, a broad range of skills and an ability to make complex judgements when faced with multiple considerations (e.g., a patient with diabetes and asthma who does not adhere to medication because they are depressed and sees no point in living to an old age and whose breathing is made worse by poor housing). These healthcare professionals need to have a sophisticated understanding about the relationship between these physical, psychological and social factors as they make decisions about diagnosis and treatment and have an attitude that focuses on the overall needs of the patient rather than on abstract notions of ideal disease control.

Training doctors and nurses

In training doctors and nurses, more recognition needs to be given to the fact that most patients they see will have multimorbidity rather than a single disease. Students need to learn more about the key factors highlighted by the chronic care model, such as promoting patient self-management (rather than assuming that doctors make decisions and patients do as they are told), the need for individual accountability in coordinating the care of complex patients and the importance of organizational factors such as recall and reminder systems. Most importantly, students need to be encouraged to develop a patient-centred attitude rather than a disease-centred attitude and an approach to consulting which is based on understanding the patient's context, sharing decisions with them and reaching an agreement about an individual management plan that reflects their priorities.

Valuing generalism

At a national level, healthcare systems need to value and promote careers that are based on generalism rather than specialism. This may be reflected in the involvement of generalist doctors in national decision-making bodies, the length of training that is deemed necessary for the role and the salaries of generalists versus specialists. In many countries, generalists earn less than specialists, and it is not surprising that in these countries it is difficult to attract the best doctors and nurses to work in generalist roles.

Planning and commissioning healthcare

Commissioners of health care seek to redesign care pathways in order to obtain the best outcomes at the lowest cost. As previously discussed, these care pathways are frequently designed on a disease-specific basis. Services are often commissioned from specific providers for an individual disease, and the performance of these providers is often monitored in terms of disease-specific targets. This can again lead to fragmentation of care. Therefore, when planning and commissioning services for individual diseases, it is important to ensure that providers can as far as possible manage common comorbidities without cross-referral and that they can communicate information effectively with the primary care professional who is coordinating the patients' overall care.

Clinical guidelines

In most developed countries, guidelines have been developed for the management of chronic diseases. The authors of guidelines need to be explicit about the extent to which these are valid for patients with comorbidities. In some cases, there may be little or no evidence about the management of patients with comorbidities on which to base guidance. It cannot be assumed that interventions are equally beneficial in patients with comorbidities as in those without. For example, a patient with cancer or heart failure has a reduced life expectancy and may have less to gain from interventions that are designed to increase their life span but at the expense of drug side-effects in the short term.

On the other hand, in the absence of evidence from patients with multimorbidity, guidelines based on patients with a single condition may be all we have to go on. It is arguable that the benefits of treatment may be even greater in patients with multimorbidity because they are at a greater absolute risk of adverse consequences of disease and therefore have most to gain from interventions.

The solution to this dilemma is not necessarily a nihilistic rejection of guidelines. Instead, it may mean that we need more sophisticated guidelines and targets that carefully define the target population and take account of comorbidities. For example, blood pressure targets may need to be more relaxed for patients who have a reduced life expectancy due to a non-cardiovascular condition but conversely more strict for patients with other conditions such as renal or eye disease, which are more progressive in patients with uncontrolled hypertension. These patient-specific guidelines should be combined with decision aids to inform management decisions that reflect the evidence and also the individual patient's preferences and needs (Figure 11.3). It is important to allow professionals to exclude individual patients from targets when there are particular reasons why achieving the target may be inappropriate or impossible; for example, because the patient makes an informed choice not to follow the guidance.

New approaches to research are needed

Guidance is at least partly based on research evidence, but much research that underpins guidelines excludes or fails to take account

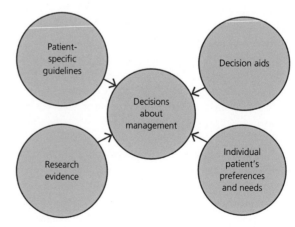

Figure 11.3 Factors that should be fed into treatment decisions about individual patients.

of patients with multimorbidity. There are clear parallels with research which in the past routinely excluded patients aged over 75, yet the findings were used to make decisions about the care of elderly patients. In future, research on interventions should include the broad range of patients to whom they are likely to be applied, including those with multimorbidity. There should be an explicit plan to compare the effectiveness of the intervention in patients with and without comorbidities. This will inevitably make trials larger and more costly as they will need to be more inclusive and large enough to allow for subgroup analysis. For research that is already published, the problem may be addressed to a degree by meta-analysis using individual patient data in order to identify subgroups with specific types of multimorbidity (e.g., particular combinations of conditions, patients with poor general health, etc.). Where patients with comorbidities are excluded from studies, more attention should be given to the serious limitation that this places on the generalizability of the research findings (Box 11.3).

Box 11.3 **Recommendations for research**

- Do not exclude patients with comorbidities from research studies
- In studies of interventions, include in the analysis plan a comparison of effectiveness in patients with or without comorbidities
- Undertake meta-analyses using individual patient data from existing trials in order to explore the impact of interventions for subgroups of patients with different types of multimorbidity
- Develop better measures of continuity and coordination of care in order to be able to assess the benefits of different approaches to delivering care
- Test organizational interventions that are designed to promote continuity and coordination of care for people with multimorbidity

---

Further reading

Bayliss, E., Edwards, A., Steiner, J. *et al.* (2008) Processes of care desired by elderly patients with multimorbidities. *Family Practice*, **25** (4), 287–293.

Epping-Jordan, J.E., Pruitt, S.D., Bengoa, R. *et al.* (2004) Improving the quality of health care for chronic conditions. *Quality and Safety in Health Care*, **13** (4), 299–305.

Hill, A.P. & Freeman, G.K. (2011) *Promoting Continuity of Care in General Practice*. Royal College of General Practitioners, London.

Salisbury, C. (2012) Multimorbidity: redesigning health care for people who use it. *The Lancet*, **380** (9836), 7–9.

Salisbury, C., Johnson, L., Purdy, S. *et al.* (2011) Epidemiology and impact of multimorbidity in primary care: a retrospective cohort study. *British Journal of General Practice*, **61** (582), e12–e21.

Salisbury, C. *et al.* (2013) The content of general practice consultations: cross-sectional study based on video recordings. *British Journal of General Practice*, **63** (616), e751–e759.

CHAPTER 12

Optimizing Outcomes in Multimorbidity

Stewart W. Mercer[1], Martin Fortin[2], and Chris Salisbury[3]

[1]General Practice and Primary Care, Institute of Health and Wellbeing, University of Glasgow, UK
[2]Family Medicine Department, Université de Sherbrooke, Centre de Santé et de Services Sociaux de Chicoutimi, Canada
[3]Centre for Academic Primary Care, NIHR School for Primary Care Research, School of Social and Community Medicine, University of Bristol, UK

OVERVIEW

- This chapter draws together the main issues arising from each chapter into an overall summary
- 'Top tips' for the practical management of patients with multimorbidity are given
- There is an urgent need for research that includes and focuses on multimorbid patients and we need both cohort studies and intervention studies
- There is a need to embed multimorbidity within medical education at undergraduate and postgraduate levels and within healthcare training in general
- Policy priorities should focus on the delivery of patient-centred care in multimorbidity
- Both research and policy should use process and outcomes measures that reflect the views and needs of patients with multimorbidity.

The story so far

In this book, we have tried to describe and discuss the key issues in multimorbidity. We have explained the ways in which multimorbidity can be defined and measured (Chapter 1), and how this influences estimates of prevalence. However measured, multimorbidity is common and likely to become more prevalent as populations age (Chapter 2). In people with long-term conditions, multimorbidity is the norm rather than the exception, and the wide range of combinations of conditions that exist challenges the current single-disease paradigm.

Multimorbidity is not just a problem of old age, and more people below the age of 65 have multimorbidity than those aged 65 years and over. This is because of the population demographics at present. Multimorbidity is socially patterned, being common in areas of higher socioeconomic deprivation. It also occurs 10–15 years earlier in the poorest communities than when compared with the most affluent in society (Chapter 2).

Multimorbidity has profound effects on quantity and quality of life, impacting negatively on functional status and quality of life (Chapter 3). It is associated with huge healthcare costs in both primary and secondary care due to higher consultation rates, more frequent hospital admissions and increased duration of stay (Chapter 4).

Primary care clinics are not well organized for the care of multimorbid patients who can seem like square pegs in round holes. There are issues of identification, continuity of care and polypharmacy resulting from the indiscriminate use of single-disease guidelines and protocol-driven consultations (Chapter 5). More than any other group, multimorbid patients require a holistic, patient-centred care tailored to the needs of the individual not their diseases (Chapter 6).

Current IT systems including the medical record are woefully inadequate in capturing and communicating the data required to enhance the care of patients with multimorbidity (Chapter 7). In addition to the substantial illness burden that multimorbidity carries, there is often a substantial treatment burden as well, due to fragmented, uncoordinated care and polypharmacy (Chapter 8). Multimorbidity is not just about physical health, and mental and physical health problems commonly coexist (Chapter 9). Mental health problems can lead on to multiple physical conditions, and multimorbidity of physical conditions can lead to mental health problems.

Multimorbidity has implications for the quality and safety, although these implications are not well understood as yet (Chapter 10). There are major policy implications for all countries regarding the funding, organization and delivery of health care to address the needs of patients with multimorbidity who are the biggest users of healthcare services (Chapter 11).

Top tips in the management of multimorbidity for clinicians

Below, we list some tips to help clinicians in their management of patients with multimorbidity (see also Figure 12.1). These tips have been distilled from the previous chapters of this book and are a list of issues that all clinicians should consider when managing patients with multimorbidity.

ABC of Multimorbidity, First Edition.
Edited by Stewart W. Mercer, Chris Salisbury and Martin Fortin.
© 2014 John Wiley & Sons, Ltd. Published 2014 by John Wiley & Sons, Ltd.

9 Maximize continuity of care, ensuring that each patient has a doctor who is clearly responsible for them.

10 Integrate the work of GPs and practice nurses in managing patients with multimorbidty; for example, by carrying out shared annual reviews (e.g., a medical review by the doctor including polypharmacy, at the end of a holistic assessement by the nurse of the patients' lifestyle, priorities and self-management goals).

Research into multimorbidity

There is a dearth of research on multimorbidity and much of the research that exists and has been referred to in this book comes from cross-sectional descriptive studies. An important precursor to developing effective interventions is detailed understanding of the development and effects of multimorbidity over time. Prospective cohort studies are the most robust observational method available for providing this because they usually have fewer potential sources of bias than retrospective and case-control studies. As alluded to in Chapter 2, we know relatively little about the trajectory and natural history of multimorbidity over time, with a recent systematic review finding very few longitudinal studies (France *et al.* 2012). Randomized controlled trials including economic analysis are also needed to provide strong evidence about cost-effectiveness, although these may be difficult to conduct. However, there is also very limited information on interventions to enhance outcomes in multimorbid patients. A recent systematic review of interventions in primary care for multimorbid patients found only 10 randomized controlled trials studies worldwide. There was a lack of studies that took into account the patients' socioeconomic status, and most studies found no evidence of benefit from the interventions tested. Clearly, a lot more research is needed!

Multimorbidity and healthcare training

There is also a lack of focus in medical education on multimorbidity both at undergraduate and postgraduate levels in many countries despite the importance of this topic. General practitioners play a key role in the management of multimorbidity, yet training for primary medical care is typically shorter than training for specialists. Indeed, many countries around the world still have no requirement for compulsory training in general practice.

Policy and multimorbidity

Policy should focus on developing and delivering real patient-centred care in multimorbidity, given the many challenges that such patients face in daily life. Health services should be at their best where they are needed most, yet the continued existence of the 'inverse care law' means that even in countries with a national health service, the multimorbid patients with greatest need continue to receive suboptimal care. Research needs to be better aligned and integrated with policy so that interventions that deliver better care, using measures that are meaningful to people with multimorbidity, can be rapidly developed and embedded into healthcare systems.

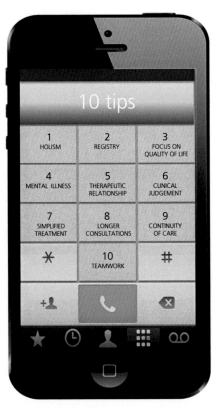

Figure 12.1 Ten top tips for the management of patients with multimorbidity. Created by Tarek Bouhali.

1 Think holism. Diseases cannot be understood outside the context of the patient who suffers from them, and it is necessary to consider the coexisting physical conditions of each patient as well as their mental health and social circumstances.

2 Have a means of identifying the patients with multimorbidity in your practice; this is likely to involve some development of electronic medical records systems.

3 Focus on quality of life rather than just indicators of disease control. For patients, improving their quality of life in the present may be more important than seeking longer life in the future, and this means they have to incur an excess treatment burden from medication or other medical interventions

4 Diagnose and treat mental illness as depression is particularly common in multimorbidity, is often under-recognized and is associated with poor outcomes.

5 Develop a therapeutic relationship through continuity of care and through developing effective consultation skills.

6 Be confident to use clinical judgement rather than slavishly following guidelines, which may not be appropriate for the patient in front of you.

7 Tackle polypharmacy by simplifying treatment regimes, using medication aids to promote adherence, ensuring that patients understand their treatments and stopping prescriptions of treatments of limited value.

8 Consider longer consultations specifically for this group of patients either by always offering them more time or allowing more flexibility in the appointment system.

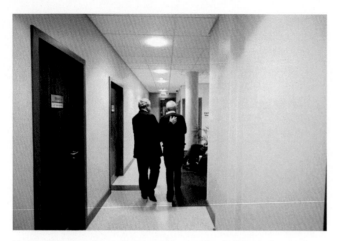

Figure 12.2 Empathic, patient-centred care will remain the hallmark of quality in the management of patients with multimorbidity.

Conclusions

Multimorbidity is now a common fact of life, yet there is a dearth of research on how to manage patients with multimorbidity, and guidelines are based on evidence that largely excludes such patients. The science no longer fits the population and the science must change. Medicine though will always remain an art and a science, and clinicians will continue to need to use – in addition to meaningful evidence – clinical wisdom, compassion and insight in order to deliver patient-centred care to this group of patients (Figure 12.2).

Further reading

France, E.F., Wyke, S., Gunn, J.M., Mair, F., McLean, G. & Mercer, S.W. (2012) A systematic review of prospective cohort studies of multimorbidity in primary care. *British Journal of General Practice*, **62** (597), e297–e307.

Smith, S.M., Soubhi, H., Fortin, M., Hudon, C. & O'Dowd, T. (2012) Managing patients with multimorbidity: systematic review of interventions in primary care and community settings. *British Medical Journal*, **345**, e5205.

Index

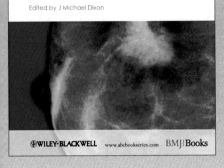

ABC of Breast Diseases

4TH EDITION

J. Michael Dixon
Western General Hospital, Edinburgh, UK

Breast diseases are common and often encountered by health professionals in primary care. While the incidence of breast cancer is increasing, earlier detection and improved treatments are helping to reduce breast cancer mortality. The *ABC of Breast Diseases, 4th Edition*:

- Provides comprehensive guidance to the assessment of symptoms, how to manage common breast conditions and guidelines on referral
- Covers congenital problems, breast infection and mastalgia, before addressing the epidemiology, prevention, screening and diagnosis of breast cancer and outlines the treatment and management options for breast cancer within different groups
- Includes new chapters on the genetics, prevention, management of high risk women and the psychological aspects of breast diseases
- Is ideal for GPs, family physicians, practice nurses and breast care nurses as well as for surgeons and oncologists both in training and recently qualified as well as medical students

AUGUST 2012 | 9781444337969 | 168 PAGES | £27.99/US$46.95/€35.90/AU$52.95

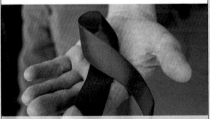

ABC of HIV and AIDS

6TH EDITION

Michael W. Adler, Simon G. Edwards, Robert F. Miller, Gulshan Sethi & Ian Williams
University College London Medical School; Mortimer Market Centre, London; University College London; St Thomas' Hospital, London Medical School; University College London Medical School

Since the previous edition, big advances have been made in treatment, knowledge of the disease and epidemiology. The problem of AIDS in developing countries has become a major political and humanitarian issue.

- Edited by the Director of the Department for Sexually Transmitted Diseases, *ABC of HIV and AIDS, 6th Edition* is an authoritative guide to the epidemiology, incidence, and most up to date management of HIV and AIDS
- Reflects the constantly changing knowledge of the disease and its manifestations, new developments in drug and non-drug management, sociological and political issues
- Includes 6 new chapters on conditions associated with AIDS and further concentration on the community effects of the disease, and the situation of women with AIDS
- Ideal for all levels of health care workers caring for HIV and AIDS patients

JUNE 2012 | 9781405157001 | 144 PAGES | £24.99/US$49.95/€32.90/AU$47.95